W9-ATZ-161

The pup wasn't much more than two weeks old, his eyes barely open. He was brown and white, of uncertain ancestry, and very, very thin. His left hind leg was mangled. . . .

We got a lot of stray animals brought in to the emergency clinic, and the outcome depended largely on the people who brought them in. If no one was willing to pay this pup's bills and offer it a permanent home, it would have to be put to sleep. I broached the subject gently.

"Assuming this little guy pulls through, are you willing to give him a home?"

I still recall Mr. Henneke's exact words: "My dear young lady, we have just spent the last eighteen hours driving nine hundred miles from La Paz, Mexico, to get this little puppy some medical care. I *think* we're going to keep him! . . ."

By Lillian M. Roberts
Published by Fawcett Books:

RIDING FOR A FALL
THE HAND THAT FEEDS YOU
ALMOST HUMAN
EMERGENCY VET

Books published by The Ballantine Publishing Group
are available at quantity discounts on bulk purchases
for premium, educational, fund-raising, and special
sales use. For details, please call 1-800-733-3000.

EMERGENCY VET

Lillian M. Roberts

FAWCETT GOLD MEDAL • NEW YORK

Sale of this book without a front cover may be unauthorized. If this book is coverless, it may have been reported to the publisher as "unsold or destroyed" and neither the author nor the publisher may have received payment for it.

A Fawcett Gold Medal Book
Published by The Ballantine Publishing Group
Copyright © 1998 by Lillian M. Roberts

All rights reserved under International and Pan-American Copyright Conventions. Published in the United States by The Ballantine Publishing Group, a division of Random House, Inc., New York, and simultaneously in Canada by Random House of Canada Limited, Toronto.

http://www.randomhouse.com

Library of Congress Catalog Card Number: 98-96102

ISBN 0-449-00043-5

Manufactured in the United States of America

First Edition: November 1998

10   9   8   7   6   5   4   3   2   1

This book is for Missouri's College of Veterinary Medicine Class of 1987.

And for all those veterinarians out there who still "do it all night long." You know who you are.

The following stories are all essentially true. They are told from memory, and due to the inherent subjectiveness of memory may have inadvertently been embellished, or details altered. Likewise, if you asked others who were present at the time, they may remember things differently. For this reason, and because many of the cases are old and the records have been purged, I have changed certain identifying factors, as well as the names of most of the clients and animals involved. In certain cases, such as where the events are a matter of public record, I have used real names. In addition, wherever possible I have used the actual names of the doctors, staff members, and referring veterinarians with whom I worked for nearly eight years. Where that is true, I have done my best to portray everyone in the best possible light. However, if anyone finds this portrayal in any way objectionable, it is the fault of the author alone, and not the editor or the publisher.

Table of Contents

Contents

*All In
A Day's Work*

The dog can barely walk when she arrives. We manage to get her into the back room before she collapses. I know at a glance what's wrong, and what to do about it. But that's only the first step.

Sheba is a six-year-old shepherd mix. Still young, basically healthy before tonight. Now she has a gastric dilatation-volvulus, or GDV: her stomach has flipped inside her abdomen, probably taking her spleen with it. Distressed and trying without success to vomit the huge meal and gallon or so of water that precipitated the crisis, she swallows air and her distended stomach seems to swell before my eyes.

The condition is fatal if not treated. To survive she must have immediate surgical correction. But surgery is only a small part of the management of such cases—the syndrome sets off a cascade of circulatory failure leading to shock, heart arrhythmias, tissue death and organ failure that must be addressed. In short, we must treat the patient and not the illness. It gets expensive, often a few thousand dollars, and a ballpark estimate was the best I could do—each case evolves uniquely. And despite all we have learned about the condition since I graduated from veterinary school, I cannot guarantee Sheba will survive this.

I have a short but uncertain amount of time to convince her owner of the urgency of Sheba's situation and get her to make a decision. First, I must prove the dog has what I think she has—a simple X-ray does that. Then I have to explain it to a distraught owner whom I have never met before, and assess her philosophical and financial commitment to her pet at a time of great distress, without offending her. She must reach a decision: surgery or euthanasia. And she must do it now.

"Please save her, I'll come up with the money somehow"

will not be good enough—she has to prove she can afford this. A substantial deposit is required.

An honest prognosis she can understand—my job. I explain. I point to the X-ray. To Sheba's belly. I show her the dog's gums, which are dry and a musty blue-gray color. They should be pink and moist. I explain some more.

"Can I call my regular vet?"

A glance at the wall clock—eleven at night. Her vet has insisted we not call him at home. "No, I'm sorry. Unless you have his home number." She doesn't.

Wavering. Lots of questions. No time to answer, to discuss the crisis in calm and dispassionate terms. "Yes or no? We'll talk about the details after."

"How much money? Can I make payments?"

Leaning toward "yes." Get an IV in. Sheba, fortunately, is easy to work on. Sharon gets a bag of fluids running, treating the shock while we decide.

"Can it happen again?"

"Almost certainly not. We'll sew the stomach to a rib."

"I don't want her to suffer."

Leaning toward "no." Put a hold on the blood work.

"She's suffering now. We can treat pain. Be sure you're making your decision for the right reasons." Left unsaid: The only real reason not to go forward is the cost. But that's a fair and valid reason.

"She's my baby. If she's going to live, I want her to."

"She's got a good chance, but I can't promise anything. A lot of it is up to her." And my clinical judgment. The decisions I make at every step. She can't know how few GDVs we see, how few veterinarians feel comfortable treating them. How new graduate vets break out in cold sweat at the mere thought. What has been tried, and has succeeded or failed, in that learning process. All the mistakes that have been made, by me and others; all that I don't know.

Leaning toward "yes." "Let's get an ECG." The tracing is nearly—but not quite—normal. This is a good sign. But the occasional ectopic beat of Sheba's heart signifies trouble coming. *Decide, decide.*

"She's had a liter of fluids. Each bag costs money. Shall I start another?"

Yes.

Sharon does it. My head tech, calm and efficient.

"The next step is to get some of the gas off, let blood circulate to the stomach again."

"Do it."

I shave a spot over the drumlike belly, scrub it briefly. Half a dozen huge needles aren't even noticed by my patient. A rush of foul gas. Whiff of Chinese food. Dog kibble. Bile.

Sheba relaxes visibly. Her breathing comes easier.

"She looks so much better. Are you sure she needs the operation?"

"The gas will come back. Sorry, but you really need to decide."

"What are her chances?" For the seventh or eighth time.

"So far everything looks good. Most of them make it." But for all I know the whole stomach will be black when I get in there. We might have to put her down on the table. Or she might never wake up from the anesthesia. Or her heart might deteriorate despite everything we can do. "There are a lot of potential complications. Too many to discuss in detail now. This pamphlet might help you understand."

"Can I make a phone call?"

"Of course. Shall I continue working on her?"

Leaning toward "yes." Run the blood work—all her organs seem to be doing their jobs. A good sign. More PVCs on the ECG—not good. Lidocaine in her IV drip. Get the OR ready just in case. Packs come out, gowns and gloves and hats and masks. What suture material? Grab some ought Vicryl. No, make it number one instead. But don't actually open anything yet—we haven't made a decision. We've spent over three hundred dollars already, and I know if the client decides now to put her dog to sleep there will be resentment over that. But I'm hoping she goes forward. I'm ready if she does. It's been a quiet night and I'm glad for something to do. Saving them is more fun than not saving them.

The buzzer, up front. Another animal has come in. Snake bite? Why didn't they call? The phone rings. Jane gets it, in another room. A cat on its way, hit by a car. They don't know if he'll make it.

They never do. That's my job.

Come on, what will it be? I'm no longer as excited about the surgery. Owner still on the phone, trying to borrow a credit card from someone—her mother?

I enter the exam room. Oscar, a black Lab puppy, couldn't resist a crackly noise, and shoved his nose into a crevice. The snake—a young one by the closeness of the punctures—nailed him on the left side of his muzzle, just behind the nose. The left side of his face is already swollen to twice its normal size. Oscar is miserable, but can't rest his head on the table. It hurts too much.

"Do what you gotta do, Doc."

It takes me a minute to realize he means put the puppy to sleep. "But we can treat him so easily!"

He is surprised. "You mean he might live?"

Wondering about our GDV case, I discuss treatment options with Oscar's "dad." Trying to hurry without seeming to hurry. Money isn't the problem here; he'd just assumed snake bites were fatal. I take precious seconds to write up an estimate. Get an IV in while the antivenin takes its time dissolving. Go slow, slow— watch for allergic reaction to the serum. Dripping, seems okay.

"So what are we going to do?" To Sheba's owner.

"Um, you're so young. How many of these dogs have you treated?"

"More than anyone else in the desert." True statement. "They happen at night."

"I've never met you before. Don't take this wrong, but. . . ." A helpless tear. "This is my dog. You're telling me I have to spend thousands of dollars I don't have, or else she's going to die. How do I know you're telling me the truth?"

I shrug. I am no longer easily offended. But I have no answer for her.

She glances at the crumpled descriptive pamphlet in her hand, complete with simplistic drawings. It bears the logo of a prominent pet food manufacturer. She stares at Sheba. The dog is beginning to pant again. Her eyes reflect distress.

"I've been saving for two years for a trip to Australia," she finally says. "I have to transfer the funds. Can I pay you tomorrow?"

"We can hold a check." I'm feeling hard-nosed, but we've been ripped off too many times.

A hesitation, then a nod.

Jane has the estimate ready. They go up front. They nearly collide with the bloody cat and its owners.

The cat is obscured by a filthy blanket. He is unconscious. Black and white, I think. One eye protrudes from its socket. His palate is split down the middle, bloody froth bubbling from the nose and open mouth. Blue-white gums: shock and blood loss.

I take the bundle, place it on the table and gently unravel it. The cat's neck is extended, its breathing labored. Ribs move counter to respiratory effort—flail chest. Internal injuries without a doubt. The tail hangs limply, bloody feces caked on it and the hind legs. Spinal fracture? Bruising? Brain injury? All of the above?

My eyes meet those of the woman who handed her to me. Lank hair, bloody clothes, despair. She is already crying but now she sobs. There is little discussion. Maybe—possibly—the cat could live, but at what cost? And in what condition? In this case we'll never know.

She signs the form and I take her pet in back. He never feels the injection, but that awful desperate gasping finally stills.

Moving on. Bag the cat, get it out of the way. I'm a little relieved I don't have two critical cases to deal with. Wish I could spare time for more sympathy but my mind is on the ones I can help.

Check the puppy. Doing fine. Already more comfortable. Get some antibiotics on board before I forget. He's finished his antivenin, switch him to lactated Ringer's.

Sheba's owner comes back to say good-bye. She doesn't want to wait. She must return before eight in the morning to move Sheba to her regular vet's. I promise to call after surgery.

Jane is leaving. Her shift is over. Anita, the graveyard tech, arrives. That's how I know it's midnight. Sharon volunteers to stay for the surgery. An extra pair of hands is welcome.

Sheba does well. Her stomach is pink, the spleen easily

removed. Heart stable. I am relieved, and gratified. It was my call and I got it right.

As I start closing my incision the doorbell rings. A dog who ate snail bait. He is already seizuring. Sharon gets the Valium ready.

Just another day at the office.

What Herriot Did

I'm no James Herriot.

I read him, of course. We all did. James Alfred Wight told a charming story, and probably inspired countless young people to attempt to follow in his footsteps, career-wise. His gentle humor and compassion made me wish I could be like that.

Trouble is, nobody can. There's a reason his stories are classified as "fiction." I'm sure part of the problem is simply the difference in our times. His was an era of small villages, where hardship was a way of life but where everyone relied on each other—I believe such a time and place existed. But in Herriot's world there was no cruelty and no evil. Everyone paid their bills. The dishonest got theirs in the end. It was not so different from the worlds created in mystery fiction, which I write in what I think of as my "Other Life."

But it bears little resemblance to the world of modern veterinary practice. Technology has not, as some would claim, replaced the personal touch. But it has seriously intruded on that gut-feeling snap diagnosis. Herriot did not always claim to know what the problem was immediately, and in some cases he admitted not having a clue. Today we are expected to know. If we don't know, we are expected to be able to find out.

Herriot did not tell his readers about owners who demanded euthanasia for animals with astonishingly treatable (and preventable) conditions—broken legs, uterine infections—because in this person's mind no animal is worth the kind of money it would take to treat it.

It becomes a vicious circle, leading to burnout. In veterinary school, we are taught the very best medicine, the newest techniques, the most advanced procedures. Our first days in practice we are told the real world isn't like that. After ten people decline all diagnostic tests and ask for "them little green pills Doc put him on last time he got sick, 'bout six years ago," we begin to believe. We may stop recommending the tests, only on busy days at first, but then gradually forget to even mention them. We know the clients don't want them, you see. Eventually, we lose the ability to interpret the tests we do manage to run. One case blends into another in our minds. We get bored with the daily sameness. We become our own worst enemies.

Picture this hypothetical (but not uncommon) scene: A man brings his ten-month-old Chihuahua to the emergency clinic. It is her first trip to any vet, ever. It is two o'clock in the morning. The little dog is exhausted from prolonged unproductive attempts to deliver a litter of puppies.

Client: She's real bad, Doc. I don't think she's gonna have them pups on her own.
Doctor: How long has she been in labor?
Client: Since I left for work this morning. About seven.

That makes it nearly twenty hours.

Doctor: Do you know who the father of the puppies is?
Client: Nuh-uh. She was gone two–three days a couple months back. We figure that's when she got it. 'F I knew whose dog did it, I'd sue for child support. (He laughs out loud. The doctor offers a weak smile. She's heard this joke before.)
Doctor: She's going to need a Caesarean section.
Client: Go ahead, Doc. This little dog means the world to me. I want the best for her.
Doctor: Okay, then. We'll get an IV started, then while my technician prepares the surgery room, I'll get you a cost estimate. We'll need a deposit. . . .
Client: You'll have to send me a bill, Doc. I was so worried about her I ran out the door without my wallet.

Now, the veterinarian knows she can save this dog. And she knows the client will never pay the bill. She is faced with two choices: Allow the client to save face by pretending to believe in this fictional wallet, or refuse to do the work until she sees the color of his cash.

Before becoming outraged, think about this: In that same week, this vet has had the opportunity to treat, also without payment: one chest-trauma case, hit by a car and presented by a bystander who has no interest in adopting the animal; a cat with an abscessed wound from a fight three days previous; one unvaccinated puppy who has developed parvoviral infection; and two stray kittens with upper respiratory infections that were dumped in the clinic parking lot in a box. All salvageable, most fatal if untreated.

She also has bills amounting to forty thousand dollars a month, and that money has to come from somewhere. Edison and GTE are remarkably unsympathetic to the plight of these animals.

The veterinarian might be forgiven for declining to treat, for euthanizing the poor dog to end her misery.

However, this night has not been without tragedy. It started with a poodle, mauled beyond repair by a roving German shepherd, dead on arrival. Then a cat whose cancer had progressed to a point where her devoted owners couldn't stand her suffering another minute. "Please, we don't want to wait until our vet opens tomorrow—put her to sleep tonight. And we want our six-year-old daughter to watch, so she can learn about death."

After that, perhaps a bird whose wings had grown more than his owners realized, who flew into a ceiling fan and mangled its chest. Despite attempts to save it, the bird died of shock and blood loss. And to top things off, in came a dog whose owners didn't realize the antifreeze it drank three days ago was poisonous. Now its kidneys are destroyed and there's nothing the DVM can offer except humane euthanasia.

And bear in mind, most of us enter this profession because we *like* animals. Losing a pet is hard on the owners, but for most it is rare. We go through it on a daily basis. This vet could use the lift that saving this one would bring.

So there we sit, at two A.M. The veterinarian is exhausted, the client an irresponsible lout who may or may not think the person across the table believes his lies. (Would *you* want a vet that stupid?) Between them a tiny dog is giving up the struggle for her own life. The puppies, undoubtedly, have already died.

Doctor: I'm sorry, but our policy is to get some guarantee of payment before providing extreme forms of treatment. Can you call someone at home and get us a credit card number?

Client: We don't believe in credit cards. Everything's cash on the barrelhead. *(translation: his credit is no good.)*

Doctor: Is there someone at home who can bring your wallet down so we can get started?

Client: *(bristling)* I can't believe you'd put money above my dog's life! Can't you see she's suffering? I always pay my bills!

Doctor: I'm sure you do. *(cough)* But we've been burned too many times. If we don't get paid, we can't pay our own bills, and soon we won't be able to stay in business. I'm sorry, but you've had all day to think about this. If you don't have it, can you borrow it from someone?

Client: I can't wake my friends at this time of day! *(But waking the vet is not a problem.)*

Doctor: Well, I don't know you well enough to lend you money, myself. So what are we going to do?

Client: I can't believe this! I guess I'll just take her home and shoot her!

But he makes no move to leave. He is assuming the veterinarian's compassion is greater than his own.

At war in the veterinarian's mind are the dog's pain and the fact that she can almost certainly save it's life, battling the fact that it will be going home with this same owner, who places little value on his pet's life. He could have prevented this situation, either by having her spayed a few months ago, or by keeping her confined when she went into heat. This little dog has never received a vaccination, and chances are if she treats it now, it will return next month with parvo, or having been run over. Her owner, knowing his lies worked the first time, will again show up in the middle of the night without payment.

Weigh that against the cumulative depression of all that has transpired this same night.

And hold that up to the fact that it's two A.M. and she could be sleeping.

She offers humane euthanasia at no charge.

The man suddenly recalls he might have left his wallet in the glove compartment of his car. He produces a three hundred dollar deposit, against a total estimated bill of around five hundred. This includes spaying her, a condition of the surgery. It should be more, but the doctor is salivating at the chance to save something. The client swears he will have the balance when he picks her up the following evening. If we're lucky, he'll show up without the money. If we're unlucky, he will disappear.

It doesn't always turn out so well. And this is hardly an extreme case. I don't know any veterinarians who won't give away services occasionally, but like most people we like to pick our own charities.

Few are prepared for this harsh reality. Veterinary school does little to get us ready. The result is a dichotomy: Many of my colleagues are perceived by their clients as uncaring, due to a wall of professional detachment they erect in self-defense. Others live on the edge of poverty, because they have learned to undervalue their own services to protect themselves against the stress of cost-based euthanasia decisions. A few are so alienated by practice that they limit themselves to traveling vaccine clinics or leave the profession altogether.

But an increasing number of veterinarians have rebelled against these extremes. An entire new field has opened up—that of Veterinary Practice Management. Consultants travel the country, counseling clinic owners on economic reality. Most make more than the veterinarians they work for. Their Lesson Number One: Don't be afraid to charge for what you do.

And slowly, the public attitude is changing. The value of the human/companion-animal bond is being recognized and appreciated. Pets live increasingly indoors, are considered part of the family. Pet veterinary insurance is now a reality. Veterinarians have spearheaded the effort to educate the public about vaccinations, dental care, grooming, spaying, and neutering. Increasingly, even shelters charge for the pets they adopt out—no longer is the animal "free" and therefore without value.

I am privileged to have graduated at a time when disposable income is at an all-time high. Luxuries such as well-cared-for pets are considered the norm. At the same time, advances in medical technology have made the profession incredibly rewarding.

In many ways, my presence both in small animal medicine and in the desert where I practice was accidental. The road to where I am has been an exciting adventure—perhaps it would not have mattered where I wound up. But I do recognize how special my situation is, how much my clients care about their pets. I realize this is not necessarily the norm.

When I read back through Herriot—ether as an anesthetic, foul and mysterious concoctions in glass syringes, the days before antibiotics were discovered—I feel mostly gratitude that I live now instead of then. I am able to enjoy his stories for what they are.

I hope you, the reader, can enjoy mine as well.

The Impossible Dream

I didn't always plan to become a veterinarian.

I especially didn't plan to become a small-animal vet.

But now I wouldn't change a thing.

I remember well the day I made the decision. I was working in Ruidoso, New Mexico, at the quarter-horse race track. It was my third summer there, and I was grooming for H. Don Farris, one of the best trainers ever to grace the profession. I was twenty-one years old, a high-school dropout who'd been horse-crazy since the day I first realized this world held such creatures. I loved my job and respected my boss.

But I couldn't afford a place to live. I worked seven days a week, seven hours (at least) per day, and I couldn't pay rent. I slept in my Chevy pickup in Lincoln National Forest, showering at the track, and thinking maybe this wasn't a career after all. The romance of nomadic existence paled in the day-to-day drudgery of doing the work and living the life.

That day it rained. Actually, it rained almost every day in Ruidoso, but that day it poured. I'd just finished morning chores and stopped at a phone booth for my monthly check-in call—collect—to my mother, who lived in Kansas City at the time. I told her I was thinking of applying for a veterinary technician program I'd heard about, in Colorado. I didn't know any details, didn't really know I'd been thinking about it until the words were out.

My mother, ever the optimist, said, "Why don't you go to vet school?"

I said, "Okay."

About then the sun peeked out and lit up the mountains that

dominated Ruidoso's landscape. It really was a gorgeous place to live.

But how did a twenty-one-year-old high-school dropout think she was going to get into vet school? It looked as if I had some work ahead of me.

The town's tiny library yielded some basic information about colleges and universities, so I wrote letters. I had never before bothered to find out what these institutions required—I had never planned to attend. Always hardheaded, I left school in Kansas after my junior year, aced the GED a year later, and joined the Army. That little adventure taught me how to drive a "real" truck, and landed me in New Jersey. I got a job walking "hots"—horses that had been to the track for their morning exercise—in the frigid shedrows of the burned-out Garden State Racetrack, which acted as a training center before the new grandstands were constructed. I was eighteen at the time, and glad for those ugly combat boots, as my other pair was literally falling apart. Snow and slush in my worn-out cowboy boots made for difficult walking. The job paid sixty-five dollars per week.

But I loved the racing atmosphere. It was filled with colorful characters from all over who drank coffee in the morning, sometimes with a splash of bourbon. Who talked about gambling as much as they did horses, and for the most part lived in the men-only dorms there on the grounds. The only other woman in the barn was a groom. I think her name was Lisa. She wanted to be a jockey. I hope she made it.

That February I moved back to Kansas City, driving west during the worst winter in anyone's memory, 1978. I drove straight through, and it snowed the whole way. In places there were more cars at odd angles in the ditches by the highway than were on the road. Many times I found myself staring up at the minuscule taillights of a semi I hadn't suspected of being there until I was five feet behind it. I later learned that long stretches of I-70 in Ohio, Indiana, and Illinois were closed the next day, and supplies airlifted in. It was the kind of blizzard that could bury a car, but those of us still moving didn't dare stop to help for fear of being stranded ourselves. I still feel guilty about the people I must have passed by, though I never saw anyone at all. Just the cars.

In Kansas City I lived at my mother's. My father, with whom I had lived since I was thirteen, had remarried while I was away, and bought a house with his new wife. There was no extra room. My relationship with my mother had been rocky for years, and her three-room cabin north of the city was cramped with my brother, then seventeen, my mother, and her fiancé, Richard. But there was land—two and a half acres, with horses and a series of runt pigs (OB-1-K'nobie; R-2 and D-2)—which were raised on leftovers and taken to slaughter when the freezer was empty. I slept on a sofa and worked at a saddlebred farm and learned to genuinely hate winter. But there were good aspects. I grew to love my mom and Richard even as I plotted my escape.

My first summer in Ruidoso was in 1978. The mountains of New Mexico enchanted me. This racing was different—more flash, less grit. The entire three-month meet was a buildup for the All-American Futurity, the largest jewel in the Quarter Horse Triple Crown. At the time it was the richest horse race in the world.

Naively, I'd headed west with little idea of what awaited. I did not know when the race meet opened, and arrived weeks early. Luckily I found a job right away—two jobs, in fact. One "local," an elderly man named Jack who owned a few horses and stabled them at a training center near the still-dormant track, hired me for ten dollars a day—seventy per week—to feed them and clean their stalls and walk them. I was thrilled to learn that, instead of the drudgery of hand-walking, out here they had machines like inverted lazy Susans, with long arms and dangling ropes, that led the horses around in wide circles.

Jack had a sixteen-year-old granddaughter whom he refused to allow to hang around with me. Race trackers, he told her, were a bad influence. Of course she hung around at every opportunity. I'm afraid she must have been greatly disappointed.

My other job was at the Roadrunner Cafe at the Thunderbird Inn, a big hotel south of town. (I may misremember the name.) First I helped refurbish it for the new owners, staining wood and painting and moving in tables. Once they opened I waited tables. I took the graveyard shift, which ended at six, enabling me to get to my other job.

Then the horsemen began arriving. In long, gaudy trailers that matched the elaborate trucks that towed them, they came. They traveled from Texas and California, from Kansas and Oklahoma and from Sunland Park near El Paso, on the New Mexico side where racing took place all winter. I would later discover Sunland Park to be a dirty, miserable place, but at the time it sounded impossibly exotic.

Illegal Mexican immigrants worked in most barns. They worked for less than I had made walking hots in New Jersey. But the threat of Immigration sweeps led the trainers to keep people like me on staff as well, even though they had to pay us twice as much and we didn't sleep in tack rooms in the barn. I was hired by Roger Fagan, a young trainer from Del Rio, Texas. I worked for him all summer, learning about horses and racing, and about the people I had chosen to surround myself with.

I slept in my truck in Lincoln National Forest for three weeks. Every morning the towering peak of Sierra Blanca greeted me when I awoke. It was an adventure. It was the summer I turned nineteen.

Then there ensued over two years of travel, of unpredictable housing, of short-term jobs. Some people worked for the same trainer for years, and I came to envy them. Most wore the lofty title "Assistant Trainer." It took me a while to catch on to the fact that, virtually without exception, these were men.

So came the day, my third summer in Ruidoso, when I stood in that phone booth in the rain and realized I had gone as far as I could at that time and place. I was as good a groom as one could be—which is akin to being an excellent cashier or a top-ranked waiter. Except those jobs probably paid better. I was proud of my ability and the tiny respect it engendered, but cognizant of the fact that this in no way prepared me for medical school.

After my conversation with my mother, I approached my employer at the time to see what he thought. H. Don Farris was a man I respected deeply, and feared slightly, in the way young employees fear their bosses. It was a quiet afternoon, not a race day, in late July. The mountains looked down upon us; for once it did not rain.

Don talked for an hour or more, and I mostly listened. Not

once did he sneer or question my chances. "It's what I'd do if I was your age," he said. And I think he meant it.

I told him I would be leaving when the meet ended.

Looking Like
A Hero

There's a truism among the non-Spanish-speaking vets here in the desert: "Buenos dias means 'hello,' adios means 'good–bye,' and Chiquita means 'female Chihuahua.' "

This Chiquita was tiny. Nine weeks old, weighing no more than a pound, she lay limply in her owner's hands when I saw her for the first time. It was a Saturday afternoon, and this was my first case of the day. I asked a few questions, eliciting the information that Tina and Emilio had changed her food the day before, and she hadn't eaten much of it.

Tina handed me the nearly weightless puppy. I checked her over: slow heart rate, low body temperature of 97 degrees Fahrenheit, very slight dehydration, pale gums, and absolutely nothing else of note.

I opened my mouth to ask whether she'd done any vomiting, any coughing, *anything* that might help me understand why she was in a coma, when according to her owners she'd been her usual pesky self that same morning.

Beneath my hand, Chiquita's heart stopped beating. It just stopped.

I muttered, "Oh, shit," and ran back to the treatment room. Thinking, *What do I do now?* I had worked at the emergency clinic only a few weeks, and this was my first arrest. As I ran I tried to formulate a plan: epinephrine to stimulate the heart, dopram for breathing. *Oh, God, how much do you give a puppy that only weighs a pound?*

I was saved from having to decide. Because oddly, her heart started beating again. I hadn't given her any drugs at all, but her heart spontaneously lurched beneath my palm and resumed a near-normal rhythm. There was no mistake—I'd been holding her the whole time. First it was beating, then it was not, now it was beating again.

How do you explain that to a distraught owner?

Unfortunately, she did not waken from her coma.

Now that I had the little girl in back, I decided to draw a tiny sample of blood for analysis, and try to start an IV. This was problematic in a pup her size. Nowadays I would have pushed a cannula directly into her bone marrow cavity, but at the time that wasn't widely done. So I slipped a needle into her jugular, drew out half a cc of blood—about what I thought she could spare—and then gave her fluids through the same needle.

To be precise, I gave her a glucose solution. Sugar, basically, in concentrated form. Because somewhere in the dim reaches of my brain I remembered learning that in diabetics, too much insulin can cause the blood sugar to drop, which leads to coma in an animal that may have appeared normal not long before. And too much insulin was not the only cause of low blood sugar, or hypoglycemia.

This little girl hadn't eaten in twenty-four hours.

My fingers, I was slightly embarrassed to note, were trembling as I administered the injection. *Slowly, slowly,* I made myself take time. Concentrated glucose can destroy blood cells if it's given too fast, and I didn't want to trade one problem for another.

Chiquita was moving before I finished the shot. By the time I was done, she had to be restrained.

Within seconds, she was standing weakly. I placed her in the incubator to warm her up, offered a spoonful of chicken baby food, and watched her discover the joys of inhaling food.

Reluctant to leave my patient, I sent Gayle, the technician, to bring Tina and Emilio back. At the sight of their little puppy—essentially dead moments before, now wagging her tail and licking her lips, in fact beginning to whine—Tina burst into tears.

I was ready to cry myself. This had been a close call.

Chiquita's recovery continued uneventfully. Analysis of the blood sample confirmed that her glucose, which should have measured in the range of 100 milligrams per deciliter, had instead been only twenty-three. That, of course, was before the infusion of glucose.

I kept her overnight, until her temperature had climbed into the normal range. She showed no sign of relapsing and her appetite remained excellent. Tina and Emilio accepted that Chiquita was not going to eat the food they'd chosen, and took home a can of a puppy food that Chiquita had eaten readily during her hospitalization.

I learned later that hypoglycemia is common in toy-breed puppies. I've heard it mentioned by well-known specialists in front of an audience. Their tiny, underdeveloped livers simply can't store enough glycogen—the complex carbohydrate that's broken down into glucose during a fast.

I'm sure the syndrome was recognized long ago, ages before little Chiquita was carried unconscious into the Animal Emergency Clinic of the Desert, where I worked. I've seen dozens of cases since, and almost all did well. But I'd never heard of it at the time. Somehow I'd missed out on this tidbit in vet school.

And, nearly ten years later, Chiquita is still the most dramatic case of hypoglycemia and recovery that I've ever seen.

A Chicken
And Some Eggs

Some animals do well despite our best efforts not to help them. That was certainly the case for one animal I treated, reluctantly, a few weeks after accepting my new position.

I had just gotten to work when MJ, our technician/office manager at the time, said, "Do you treat chickens?" She was holding the phone against her neck.

"Not really," I said.

"There's a lady on the phone, her kid has a chicken. It sounds like it's pretty sick. Do you want to take a look at it?"

Most of what we learned about poultry in vet school involved "sacrificing" two or three from a flock, performing autopsies, and putting drugs in the water to treat the rest of the flock based on the results. But this wasn't a flock, it was one bird. I had no idea how to treat one hen.

I said, "No, I'm sorry. I wouldn't know what to do with it."

She repeated my decision into the telephone and we both assumed that was the end of that.

Not so. An hour later I walked into an exam room to see a Rhode Island Red hen named Ruby lying on the table. Behind her stood a ten-year-old boy with tears in his eyes, and next to him, his mother.

"We didn't know where else to go," she said as I entered the room. "I called four vets today and no one would see her."

I opened my mouth to tell them I knew nothing about chickens, and really didn't think I should experiment on theirs. That they could buy quite a lot of chickens for what it would cost for me to treat this one.

"It's my 4-H project," the boy explained. I hadn't known

they even had 4-H in the desert. "I'm going to be a vet when I grow up."

So I looked at his chicken. What else could I do?

Ruby was very, very sick. And she had been sick for a while. Those were my impressive clinical observations.

More specifically, Ruby's keel jutted sharply in her emaciated chest, and the skin on her feet was wrinkled from dehydration. She lay limply on the table as I silently cursed myself for getting into this situation. Stalling for time, I palpated her abdomen—empty—and listened to her lungs and heart with my stethoscope. Nothing remarkable there. I thought she had some diarrhea, but who could really say?

Finally I had to tell them something. "I don't think she's going to make it," I said. What an understatement. Birds as thin and weak as this rarely survived the night. The boy's tears trickled down his cheeks and my heart sank. "I'll do what I can."

Well, dehydration is straightforward enough. I could definitely give her some fluids. And I recalled that chickens had a lot of bacterial diseases, so antibiotics were in order. At the time we could still get a sweet-tasting liquid antibiotic called chloramphenicol palmitate, which has since been taken off the market due to lack of demand and potential side effects in humans. That's what I prescribed for Ruby. And a shot of calcium and B vitamins for good measure, because that's what I would do if the hen were a parrot, and because I suspected Ruby had not been eating much lately, and these nutrients are rapidly depleted. And I force-fed her some of the baby bird formula I used in sick parrots.

"Let me know how she does," I said as they left.

They said they would. They didn't. So I assumed Ruby had died. Nowadays I would call to find out for sure, but at the time I didn't want to make them tell me the painful news.

Two years passed. Ruby was forgotten. A family brought me a cat with a urinary obstruction, a common problem which I treated routinely by hospitalizing the cat and placing a catheter to relieve the obstruction. Before they left the woman said to me, "You don't remember us, do you?"

I had to admit I didn't.

"We brought you a chicken a couple of years ago."

I remembered the chicken. She's still the only one I've ever been asked to treat. Rarely have I felt so useless. I prepared for a litany of my incompetence.

"She's doing fine."

"You mean she's still alive?" I blurted.

"She's doing great!"

And when she picked her cat up the next morning to transfer to her usual vet, she brought me four eggs. Ruby's eggs. They were the best eggs I ever tasted.

Getting In,
Getting Through

Veterinary school took on an aura of mysticism. I consulted everyone I knew—especially the track vets and a student who worked for one of them and would be starting veterinary school that fall. Their advice was hauntingly similar.

"You know the odds? Eight or ten applicants for every position."

"It's harder to get into than medical school."

"Don't even try if you haven't got a four-point-oh GPA."

"Check into the salaries. And remember, you'll probably have twenty thousand dollars in student loans to pay back."

It turned out to be over forty.

"Being female's an advantage," some said. "The big schools have to take a certain number of women."

"Women'll never make it in that field," someone predicted. "They can't handle the long hours. It's too physical."

The latest statistics predict women will outnumber men in the profession by the year 2004.

As usual, I listened but turned the advice around to suit my needs. I'd worry about the odds later. I already knew I could handle the hours and the work. The salaries they mentioned were worlds above anything I'd ever made before. Others had loans, why should I be different? And if I needed a straight-A average, then that's what I would have.

But first, there was the small matter of getting into and through undergraduate work.

I soon learned that, since I was over twenty-one, I would not be required to take the terrifying SAT test. Despite my indifference, my high school grades were not bad. There would be no scholarships, but with luck I wouldn't be turned away either.

Within a few months I was transformed from a young and rudderless dropout to a person whose goals extended beyond the next race meet. I don't think I really expected to make it, but having a long-term goal was such a new experience, I stuck with it. Within days of making the decision, I found a place to live, a mobile home with two roommates. This bit of luck served to subtly reinforce my plans. I got a second job, waitressing at the local Pizza Hut at night, and the money went into the bank for tuition.

That fall I moved back to Kansas City and my mother's sofa. I applied and was accepted to a small private school called Park College. I learned about Pell grants and student loans. I came too late for the fall semester, but found work at a training barn breaking young horses. That spring I took basic biology, English, a math refresher course, and statistics. I received As in each.

The following year I transferred to Arizona State. The big university was terrifying, but I was experienced in adapting. Within days of arriving, I was registered and had a place to live and a roommate who was an art major. I signed up for eighteen hours, and found inconsistent work exercising horses at a training center near Turf Paradise track, which was not yet open for the winter season. Paying rent, tuition, and my monthly truck payment became acts of faith.

Inorganic chemistry was my first major stumbling block. Surrounded by two hundred kids only a few years my junior, I stared numbly at the periodic table they all seemed so familiar with. In the first hour we had breezed through three chapters of the text I had yet to acquire. I began to realize that this class was aimed at freshmen who had taken high school chemistry the year before. The material was dry, boring, and strange. I had never learned the art of studying. I had trouble staying awake during class. Apparently I wasn't alone—by the second week, empty seats had already begun to appear.

I received a sixty on my first examination. Classwide scores overall were abysmal, but at least one person had gotten a hundred, so it was possible. I was devastated, ready to quit altogether. I watched my roommate and wondered if I could make it in the art department. I studied my paper to see where I'd gone wrong. Some of the answers were obvious—my brain had simply frozen under the pressure. Now I could either drop the class, or learn to study.

The only good news was, we were graded on a curve, and were allowed to drop our lowest test score at the end of the semester. I began sleeping with my chemistry textbook. The ninety-eight I got on the second test probably went further than anything before it to cement my belief that all things were possible.

My second year at ASU I was getting the hang of things. Joining (and acting as vice president for) the campus pre-vet club gave me access to materials about veterinary colleges around the country. This was the research I should have done earlier. I'd chosen ASU for my undergrad studies because of its proximity to a race track, and for Tempe's climate. As usual, I'd gone about things all wrong.

Undergrad was just one step. A test of sorts, a chance to develop the basic science skills I would need later but also a contest wherein students competed for slots in various postgraduate programs.

Nationwide, there was a ratio of about six applicants to every opening at a college of veterinary medicine. That was the average—for students applying from out of state, the odds were much worse.

Arizona did not have its own college of veterinary medicine. Instead, it had an agreement with several western states to accept a certain number of Arizona residents into their programs each year. The University of Arizona in Tucson was the Ag school of choice—not ASU. And I was excluded from the WICHE (Western Interstate Commission for Higher Education) program anyway, because I had never established myself as an Arizona resident.

I had the grades—a perfect four-oh going into my fourth semester at ASU. I had worked and carried a full load, proving myself able, yet it might not be enough. I'd chosen the wrong state for the wrong reasons.

My best bet—my only real chance—was to apply to a college of veterinary medicine in a state that would consider me an in-state student. That meant Missouri, where my mother lived, or Kansas, where I'd had my abbreviated high school career and where my father still resided. But both states tended to smile most benevolently upon those whose undergrad studies had been completed within the same university system.

I was only a sophomore. I could have transferred north. And I might have done so, had things worked out differently.

Early that year I had acquired a list of the prerequisites needed for acceptance into various colleges of veterinary medicine. In the case of Missouri, these did not include a bachelor's degree. In fact, with a little imagination and a fair amount of hard work, the classwork could be completed in two years. With nothing to lose, I requested and completed the voluminous application in November of my second year at Arizona State. I mailed it off and began the most nerve-wracking wait of my life.

I was summoned for an interview in February. I could not afford a plane ticket. I drove to Missouri for that meeting, taking two days off from classes to do so. The roads were familiar but treacherous.

The interview was on Saturday morning. I met the applicant before me, going out as I was ushered in. She looked both worried and relieved. I was seated at the end of a long oval table and introduced to six or seven people, the admissions committee. The questions began.

"Why did you drop out of high school?"

"What sort of income do you expect when you graduate?"

"Why do you want to be a vet?"

I can't remember anything I said in reply, except when someone asked why I had joined MENSA, I answered, "because I could." Why would anyone?

They had promised an answer by March 22. As the day drew near I found myself rushing home to check the mail each day, with a mixture of dread and anticipation. The answer arrived March 21, and I knew I had been accepted before I ever opened the bulky envelope. "I'm sorry, please try again next year" can be said in a one-page letter. This was a large envelope, a packet of materials welcoming me to the University of Missouri College of Veterinary Medicine and giving me an idea of what to prepare for.

I was in!

Veterinary School: A Journey

The information sent with that packet—the one that started with "Congratulations!"—was somewhat helpful in preparing for the first day. It discussed campus housing, the Honor Committee, a little bit about the curriculum, and a list of what the incoming student would need.

It also espoused a dress code. However, the list either had not been updated for some time, or was produced by a well-meaning but delusional faculty member. I cannot recall the exact words, but to paraphrase: "The Professional Student shall be at all times presentable and shall represent his future profession in a way so as to engender respect. Men shall wear button-down shirts and ties with dress slacks; however, jackets may be replaced with clean white laboratory coats. Women shall wear skirts or dresses or dress slacks . . ." It did not go so far as to discuss skirt length.

From day one, students wore T-shirts, jeans, shorts . . . in essence, we looked exactly like any other students on any other campus. It simply did not make sense to wear good clothes while dissecting formaldehyde-soaked cadavers or while holed up in the library desperately trying to cram information into your already overstuffed head prior to a crucial exam.

And they were all crucial.

That first day I chose a seat near the back and surveyed my new classmates: seventy-five men and women, roughly half of each. They hailed from farms, cities, and small towns. Most had spent their lives in Missouri, Nebraska or Arkansas—states whose reciprocal agreements allowed their students to attend veterinary school as in-state students. A surprising number were older than I. Were they as nervous as I?

I felt suddenly shy, intimidated by what I assumed were smarter, better-educated people. What made me think I could do this? College was one thing, but this was medical school! As one faculty member after another took the podium to explain what lay ahead, to warn us about the dangers of stress and over-achievement, my heart beat with pride and terror. I was in too far to change my mind. A four-year commitment? I'd never stuck with anything that long!

The vet school's buildings were old and mismatched. Some predated World War II. Within those halls matters of life and death were decided. Inside those walls countless students before me had learned to participate in those decisions. Here I would spend four years and emerge a changed person. If I made it. And that was far from certain.

Over the first year, we lost seven students from our starting class of seventy-six. All but one were excused due to poor grade performance. The seventh apparently decided this was not the profession for her.

Our class contained the usual mix—gunners whose primary goal was to graduate at the top of the class; students who only hoped to survive, and whose motto was C=DVM. The great hulking mass of us rested in the middle. We would go on to private practice or academia, industry or the military, highly competitive zoo practice or the rarified air of specialization, or the personal satisfaction of humane society clinics. An astonishing number of us would realize our dreams.

It was definitely a case of work hard/play hard. I sometimes recall vet school as a long string of parties. Hot tub parties, barbecues, beer bashes, the lobsterfest after we made the transition from classroom-bound sophomores to clinic-oriented juniors. There were volleyball, basketball, and Ultimate Frisbee—a game whose rules I never quite understood. After the stress of too much time in the library or the anatomy lab, we needed these activities to burn off steam.

We endured harsh winters and muggy summers together. We suffered injury and indignation, triumph and tragedy. Marriages and babies, deaths and divorces marked the passage of time. We were all in the same place, at the same time, but no two of us experienced it the same way.

In October 1997 I returned to Columbia for the first time since graduation. The facility was unrecognizable. Thanks to millions of dollars of public and private contributions, Mizzou now has a veterinary teaching hospital that defies description.

The occasion of my return was my tenth-year class reunion. I'm sure everyone feels their class was the best and brightest, but my classmates shine. It's been an interesting road, and a few classmates have, for all intents and purposes, vanished. But those I know rank among the best human beings I've ever encountered, and I am terribly proud to count myself among them.

A Hole
In His Head

I inherited Tiger's case my first day on Small Animal Medicine rotation. Because he'd come in at night, he had been placed in the ICU. Fortunately there were only one or two other animals in there at the time, so traffic was minimal.

The four-pound poodle hated me from the moment his beady little eyes first met mine. He lay curled in the far corner of his cage, and made no effort to get up when I went to examine him. As I opened the door, he pulled back his tiny upper lip and showed me what was left of his teeth.

I decided to read the chart and wait for a clinician. The chart didn't have much to tell me.

Tiger was almost four years old. He'd been presented to the emergency service at the University of Missouri Veterinary Teaching Hospital the night before, for lethargy. This had been going on for a few days, and his regular vet could not figure out what the problem was. Strictly speaking, it was not an emergency, but evening was the only time the owners could come, so the transfer was arranged.

I reached for the phone to contact Tiger's referring veterinarian. He was a mixed-animal practitioner in a farming town two hours away. He'd treated the little dog for a little over twenty-four hours before referring him.

"Can you tell me what he had before you referred him?" I asked.

"I gave him a cc of ————." He named a solution I'd never heard of.

"What's that?" I asked, embarrassed.

"It's used in cows. An IV solution, it has dexamethasone in it, and calcium, in an electrolyte base."

31

"How much dexamethasone?"

"Let me see. Ten grams in a liter."

I did some quick mental calculations. A cc, or cubic centimeter, is the same as one milliliter, or ml. "That's ten milligrams for a four-pound dog!" The correct anti-inflammatory dose would be more like half a mg.

"But I only gave him a cc!"

I realized I'd implied criticism, which was not my place as a student. "I'm sorry," I said. While this country vet was clearly out of his league dealing with ferocious poodles, at least he'd recognized that fact and sent the dog to the teaching hospital.

"Did you have a specific diagnosis in mind?"

A long silence followed and I began to hate myself. "You'll let me know what you find out?" he finally said.

I assured him we would, and hung up before I got myself in any deeper.

As it turned out, his "treatment" had probably saved the little dog's life.

My examination revealed—with little effort on my part, since Tiger was so willing to show me the inside of his mouth—a fracture of the rostral maxilla, or the part of the bone holding the upper front teeth. The break, which was pretty obvious now but probably had not been earlier, extended from one side just in front of the canine tooth, up toward the lip then sideways across the entire front of his mouth to the other canine.

When the intern, Dr. Scott Lozier, arrived, we threw a towel over Tiger and scooped him out of the cage. Our inexpert exam did not reveal anything further. Tiger went back into his cage until rounds. He immediately returned to his previous position, curled up in the far corner, snarling at anyone unwise enough to come near.

That afternoon an internist, Dr. C. B. Chastain, joined our investigation. We followed the same protocol: scooped Tiger up in a towel and restrained him on the exam table while going over him with our hands, our eyes, stethoscopes and otoscopes and thermometers and whatever instruments were handy. Everything was normal.

"Is he eating?" Dr. Chastain asked in his quiet voice, eyes on the table.

I glanced in the cage. Food and water dishes lay untouched. "No, not at all."

"Okay, get an IV in him so he doesn't get any more dehydrated than he already is. We'll probably turf him to Surgery to get that jaw fixed. But first I'd like Dr. O'Brien to have a look at him."

Dr. O'Brien was our resident neurologist. Dr. Chastain went to make the arrangements while I set up for a catheter. With the help of the ICU students—both of them—and a muzzle, I got the line in and secured it. Other than snarling at us, Tiger actually made little effort at resisting. I began to wonder if he would really hurt anyone, or if his attitude was merely self-defense. He seemed happiest with his head down and his eyes closed.

Dr. O'Brien and Dr. Chastain came in. Dr. Lozier followed. Tiger was already on the table, so I didn't have to repeat the towel procedure.

After briefly repeating our once-over, Dr. O'Brien placed Tiger on the floor. The little dog stumbled in a circle, then walked sideways, until he ran into a table leg. Then he collapsed and lay still.

"Yeah, he's neurological," Dr. O'Brien said.

We all nodded.

"He's got an open fontanelle," he said.

The intern and I exchanged glances. We'd both missed it. I wasn't even sure what one was.

I didn't have to wonder for long. Dr. O'Brien placed the dog back on the table, Tiger snapping a weak protest at being lifted. We all took turns palpating the large defect in the top of his domed skull. An open fontanelle. A hole in his head the size of the end of my thumb, where the bones should have grown together but never did.

"Chances are he's got hydrocephalus, and the increased pressure prevents the fontanelle from closing."

"But he's four years old! Wouldn't it show up before now?"

"Not necessarily. A lot of these cases are subclinical their whole lives. It's possible the stress associated with the fracture and not eating for several days caused him to decompensate."

I could not recall a mention of this in any lecture.

"What are you treating him with now?" Dr. Chastain asked.

"Nothing yet."

I explained about the dexamethasone.

"I'd go with some pred [prednisone, a steroid] and Lasix [a diuretic]." He specified exact doses.

"How do you confirm this?" I asked stupidly, still not quite believing.

"Radiology. The usual method is a pneumoventriculogram. I'll talk to Dr. Latimer and arrange it."

I had to look it up. A pneumoventriculogram is the process of injecting air into the chambers of the brain and taking radiographs, or X-rays, of the skull. The air shows up as black spaces in the monotonous gray of the brain matter. But the procedure is not without risks. Putting a needle into the brain can have severe negative consequences. I wondered if it was so important to have a definitive diagnosis. Couldn't we just treat the most likely thing and monitor the results?

But that's not how things were done in school. Even if the tests were worse than the disease, they would be done. Who was I to argue? I was there to learn.

The following morning, however, little Tiger was much better. He actually lunged at me, instead of just sitting back and threatening. And he did so without falling over.

"Great," I muttered, having mixed feelings as I threw the towel over him and scooped him out. He was catching on to this trick, and tried to nail me through the fabric. "You ought to be nice to me! I may be the only friend you've got around here!"

He was not impressed. He was, however, hungry. He ate a whole jar of baby food off a tongue depressor as I scooped it out of the jar.

I gave him his medications—both by injection, thankfully, so I didn't have to try to pill the little shark—and went off to daily clinics. Sometime during the day Radiology would come and take him away to do their procedure. I was glad I wouldn't be there to see.

Just before Rounds, Dr. Chastain handed me some photographs. They were Polaroids. It took me a few minutes to figure out what I was looking at.

"They ultrasounded him?"

Dr. Chastain, in his typical understated way, explained that yes, the brand-new ultrasound machine had been used to scan a picture of Tiger's brain. It does so with noninvasive and completely harmless sound waves, which are reflected off tissues in varying patterns depending upon their densities.

The sonogram had confirmed Tiger's hydrocephalus. It had done so without needles or injections or X-rays of any kind.

Sound waves cannot penetrate bone. Therefore, ultrasound's usefulness is limited where the brain is concerned. But in Tiger's case it worked great. They'd pointed the probe through the hole in his head—the open fontanelle.

Ultrasound was a new investigative tool at the time, in human and especially in veterinary medicine. It has opened up entire worlds of images heretofore unimagined. In Tiger's case it meant the difference between a simple, painless procedure that didn't even require anesthesia and a potentially fatal diagnostic test that no one really wanted to subject him to.

Before my eyes, medicine was changing shape. And I hadn't even graduated yet.

Tiger did fine. The loose piece of maxilla and the teeth it contained were removed by Surgery the next day. He went home a few days after that with a funny-looking smile and an odd haircut—sort of Poodle With A Flattop. And his attitude intact.

Months later, as a preceptor working in an equine hospital, I got to impress my boss by suggesting the use of his new ultrasound to diagnose the same problem in a foal. Unfortunately the foal did not fare so well. We also diagnosed a three-chambered heart in the same foal, and had the probe on its chest even as that heart stopped beating forever. Without it, we could not have documented the pointlessness of attempting to save him.

Today this tool is used routinely to image organs from the prostate to the heart, from tendons to eyes, the liver to the brain. It's expensive and requires a certain level of skill; I don't own one yet. But every time I think of buying one, each time I look at them in exhibit halls at conventions, I remember Tiger.

Four pounds of Attitude, and a hole in his head.

Getting
A Job

Like most students, I started looking for a job long before graduation. Not that jobs were hard to come by—unless one was particular.

I wanted to work with horses. It was my goal since the idea of vet school first percolated in my brain, and equine practice had been my focus all along. Sure, I'd enjoyed small animal clinics, but that was beside the point. I'd even noticed I had a certain aptitude for small animals, but it didn't matter. I was going to be an equine veterinarian. Period.

Unlike small animal practitioners, equine vets all seem to know each other. Many of the few jobs available were never advertised. So much depended on luck—hearing about the opening, finding a commonality with the practice owner, something to draw attention to oneself. References were vitally important, and to this end I'd spent every "free block" at a high-profile horse hospital, working seven days a week for no pay, or in one case $25 a week. I had the experience, I had the names, now all I needed was the right break.

I crossed the country, straining the tires on my Nissan pickup, occasionally sleeping in it. All things I'd done before, but this time there was an underlying sense of panic. What if I didn't get a job? There weren't many open—the horse market had crashed while I was in school, and the few jobs in equine practices were still more open for men than for women.

The only advantage I had was a total absence of loyalty to any one geographic location. And so I traveled.

For two months I lived out of suitcases, using my mother's farm north of Kansas City as a base. I would scan the JAVMA want ads, other journals' classifieds, call people I knew, people they knew, tracking rumors of potential jobs. After lining up as many "interviews" as possible in a geographic area, I started driving. Usually I arrived late at night, and had to impose on a potential employer for lodging. This was expected. I was hardly the only new graduate seeking employment.

For one or two days at a place, I "rode along." That is, I sat in the passenger seat while the practice owner drove from farm to farm, or house to house, to vaccinate healthy horses or treat lame ones or oil colicky ones. I displayed my knowledge and my ignorance, proved I could pull a shoe, pass a stomach tube, palpate a follicle, float teeth, hit a vein, spot a lameness, chat knowledgeably with a horse owner; smile and get along. I carried buckets of warm water, cleaned instruments, drew blood, counted tubes of wormer and filled out Coggins test forms.

And then I went home—my mother's home—and waited. I always came away with a sense of which position might truly be mine. I daydreamed about what my life would be like in Virginia or Maryland or Pennsylvania, North Carolina or Ohio or northern Illinois. I resisted the impulse to call my first choices on a daily basis, wished I lived closer so I could just show up every day until the clients knew me and the staff thought I worked there. Make myself indispensable and they'd have to hire me.

Mom had given me a mastiff puppy as a graduation gift, and I cherished the between-interview bonding time. While I was gone she stayed behind, drinking fresh goat milk and playing with the other dogs. She didn't seem to mind, but it caused me no end of guilt. I'd always avoided owning dogs because of the unpredictability of my future. Della now represented the possibility of settling. As far as she knew, this was home.

On the day after each job was supposed to have been filled, I called. Sometimes I was put off while "one more person" was interviewed. Other times, I was told the job had been given to a man—but if he hadn't come along, I'd have had the job! Sure. One man I really didn't want to work for told me my personality was too strong (whatever that means!).

These were jobs with starting salaries of between twelve and twenty thousand dollars a year. This was in 1987. New graduates lined up for these positions and frequently had to compete with those just finishing internships or with a couple of years' experience.

I spoke to other young vets who had graduated before me. I listened to horror stories of employers who abused new graduates by making them take emergency calls every night, then discarded them when they wore out. Male practice owners who made sexual advances toward female associates. People who had actually qualified for and completed prestigious residencies in equine medicine, only to work in small-animal emergency clinics because there were no jobs for people with their skills.

May passed, then June. The number of jobs dwindled. Breeding season ended, show season was well under way. I was still looking. Interviewing with mixed practices, those that served both large- and small-animal owners. Lowering my sights, telling myself it was temporary. Catching myself, refusing to let it happen.

I'd been all over the eastern half of the country. Finally I decided to move to California. It had been a difficult place to go for interviews, because I had to fly. That meant either renting a car or being picked up at the airport. It was expensive and impractical on a regular basis. But if I lived there, got to know people, I might just be at the right place when the right position came along. And it was time I started supporting myself, one way or another.

I could, after all, go back to exercising race horses. Maybe take a job as a resident vet at a small horse farm, doubling as a rider. Get established, be available when one of the larger practices needed help. I knew that many such jobs were filled without ever being advertised. So I put everything I owned into the back of my truck and headed west.

Déjà vu. On the road again, and all that crap. At least now I had friends and relatives along the way I could stay with. No more sleeping in my truck.

And I had company. The cats stayed at my mother's farm, but Della rode with me. For a puppy she was extremely tolerant of long periods of confinement, in the space behind the seats, a blanket spread out and a few chew toys at hand. I talked to her as I drove, told her about how life in California would be. She listened well and didn't comment.

The trip took a week, though of course I could have made it in less time. I enjoyed stopping to renew old acquaintances. And the uncertainty of what waited removed any sense of urgency I might have felt. But along the way, a curious thing happened. A letter came, with a job offer. Just like that.

It wasn't my dream job by any means. The word "equine" didn't appear anywhere in the description. It wasn't even in southern California, where I'd been headed. And the letter didn't catch up to me until I was in Phoenix.

I was tired and discouraged. I was nearly broke, and afraid I'd never have a chance to put my infant skills to use. Twice on the way I'd almost lost Della, once at a rest stop and again when she jumped a fence at a friend's in New Mexico. I was now in Phoenix, staying with a roommate from my undergrad days, in the same house we'd lived in in college. She had been in graduate school at the time, and was now established as a state employee with a steady income. After all that education, here I was, still crossing the country looking for a home.

I had been to veterinary conferences, spoken to small-animal practitioners who had offered me jobs on the spot. I had dismissed them out of hand. Now this letter came.

I phoned my mother from Phoenix, not knowing about it yet. She had opened the letter. She read it to me now. It seemed the San Francisco Bay Area Rotating Internship—a new program sponsored by a group of private specialty practices in northern California—had been left with an opening when one of their initial choices, a classmate of mine, had not passed the grueling California state board examination. There was no shame in that—somewhere around forty percent fail each time the test is offered. But I had passed back in February, and was licensed in the state. I'd had Small Animal Medicine with this classmate, and she'd heard I was still looking for a job. Did I want hers? She would be staying on, working as a technician until the next opportunity came to take the exam.

So I changed my route and headed north. I'd never been to northern California, and found myself wishing, as I drove, that I had time to stop and sightsee. I drove through the Sierras during the horrible fires of 1987, and through the San Joaquin Valley—farm land familiar to a girl from the Midwest, but the crops strange and exotic. Artichokes and oranges did not grow in Kansas. I arrived at my classmate's condo, got cleaned up and visited the practice for my interview.

After auditioning for positions all summer, it was a strange sensation to realize they had cleaned up Danville Veterinary Hospital to make a good impression on me. I met one of my future employers, Roger Kuhn, took a tour of the small facility, and heard a description of the internship program. It all took maybe fifteen minutes. Afterward he said, "When can you start?"

Maybe I gave up. I prefer to think of it as refocusing. I hadn't considered myself qualified to work in a "good" small-animal practice, since all my energy had been directed at horse work. So I assumed those desperate souls who offered me positions sight unseen operated primitive clinics and abused their new graduate associates by making them take all the emergency calls. Maybe they did; I never checked. But this was the first time I'd stood inside a clinic, looked around and imagined myself as part of it.

I went to work a few days later. Being surrounded by seven other new grads, I quickly realized two things: (1) I wasn't any more scared or uncertain of my own skills than anyone else, and (2) I had one heck of a lot to learn.

The Steep Side
Of The Learning Curve

The first rotation of my internship was night duty at Valley Veterinary Hospital in Walnut Creek. This had previously been a standard, daytime practice. It was the only one of the three sponsoring hospitals that was not directly overseen by a board-certified specialist of some kind. Though it was owned by Dr. Kuhn, who was a diplomate of the American Board of Veterinary Practitioners, he rarely visited the practice except during our weekly intern meetings.

In fact, the three veterinarians who worked there seemed to resent the interns' presence. Their outright scorn and patronizing attitudes carried to the technical staff, so that I quickly learned to dread going in. My shift began an hour before closing time, but I tried to arrive early. No matter what they thought of my abilities, I knew I needed to learn from them. And I was not so introverted that I couldn't understand their concern in leaving animals in the care of one so inexperienced.

So I learned to enter a record into the computer system. I learned the basics of performing a physical examination—not the forty-five-minute ordeal I'd gleaned from vet school clinics, but an efficient, systematic evaluation which could be done in about two minutes. After one or two hours' instruction, they went home and left me alone with one postoperative case and a long night ahead of me.

It was very, very quiet. Della was with me, wonderful adaptable companion that she had been, and she curled up on a blanket with a chew toy while I perused journal articles and finally resorted to a mystery novel. Some pressure—here I was alone on emergency duty, my worst fear realized, and nothing was happening.

Then, around eleven, the doorbell rang. I jumped about three feet, thinking, "If I don't answer maybe they'll go away." By then I was running, because it rang over and over again, with the urgent persistence of a true disaster on the hoof. And my mind wondered what the unknown people on the other side of that door would think if they knew how ill-equipped I was to deal with whatever it was they'd brought so anxiously. I opened the door.

"Our dog has been run over!" said a woman's frantic voice.

"Quick, I don't know if he's going to make it!" said a man's.

I took the unconscious toy poodle and cradled it in one arm, already moving toward Treatment while they followed. My other hand moved over the dog, performing the examination which was not yet automatic. Gently squeezing the chest, I imagined I could feel a faint heartbeat, but I had not seen or felt him take a breath. Part of me marveled that I had the presence of mind to do even that much.

But I pulled up short in the hallway leading to Treatment. The little dog's skull felt like a beanbag. I snatched the penlight from my pocket, shone it in each eye—nothing. The pupils were wide open and did not respond to the beam.

My heart lurched, and I felt my hands trembling slightly from the adrenaline rush. But this one was fairly obvious. I felt the chest again, realizing the heartbeat I thought I'd felt was a result of my own wishful thinking. I shook my head, scrambling for the words to tell these poor people the worst.

"There. . . . It's too la. . . . He's gone. There's nothing I can do. His skull. . . . He must have been killed instantly."

"Oh, my God," the woman wailed. I noticed her for the first time. Short, plump, ordinary. "But there's no blood! He isn't bleeding. There must be something you can do!"

The man, taller, gray-haired, wearing gray trousers and a polo shirt, put his arm around his wife and drew her close. It was an obvious effort for him to remain calm. "Are you sure?"

"Yes. Um . . . do you want to feel this?"

I knew my mistake before the words were out. He took a step back, shaking his head. I stood there, cradling these peoples' pet, feeling a crazy mix of misery and relief. The latter resulted from the knowledge that it wasn't my own lack of experience; there truly was nothing anyone could have done for this dog. But I had never had to tell someone their pet was dead. In school that was done by the doctors. Now I was the doctor.

This had been a young dog, his demise sudden and unexpected, and now a stranger was telling them it wasn't even worth the effort to try to save him. I couldn't imagine how they felt.

"His pupils are fixed and dilated," I said inanely, repeating a phrase everyone has heard on television, but which has little real meaning in veterinary medicine. Amazingly, it worked.

"He . . . he didn't suffer?" the woman said hopefully.

"No, I'm sure he didn't suffer."

We stood there a moment longer, me holding the dog, them seeming farther and farther away.

"Do you want me to keep the body?"

They glanced at each other. "What do you do with them?"

I had no idea. "I think they're cremated."

"You think?" For the first time they seemed to notice how young I was. "You don't even know?"

"We want to be sure he's cremated," the woman said. At least they had something to focus on besides their immediate grief.

"I . . . I'm new here, but I can find out if you like."

"Do that."

"Right." I glanced at the dog still in my arms, then down to the office, which held the nearest telephone but also my dog and the evidence of my earlier inactivity. Then over my shoulder toward Treatment, which seemed my best bet. As expected, the couple followed me there.

It was a relief to lay the tiny body on the treatment table. I picked up the phone and speed-dialed one of the other sponsoring clinics, and asked another intern what was done with the bodies. Such a mundane question, one I felt I should have known the answer to. I learned that they were, indeed, cremated by the local humane society. I passed the information along to the couple, whose names I hadn't even learned. While on the phone, I asked what I should do about charges, since I didn't feel I'd done anything.

This is the one place where new graduates hesitate most. We do not value our own services, and could not afford them ourselves if the roles were reversed. Thus, we have a tendency to undercharge for our work. However, if the clients do not pay the practice, the practice cannot pay its veterinarians, and we make even less.

During the day, this aspect of the practice was handled by the receptionists. Tonight I was on my own. I had a choice between leaving the dog's body on the table, or wrapping it in plastic and putting it in the freezer while they watched. I placed a towel over it and left it for the moment. The clients said their last good-byes and followed me up front.

Fortunately, these were clients of the practice, so they already had a file. It was a simple thing to enter the fees into the computer. I felt like a louse handing these grieving people a bill under the circumstances.

Grimly, the man wrote out a check for the emergency visit and cremation, and I handed him a receipt. I offered final condolences for their loss and escorted them out the door.

My first case was over.

To Smell A Rat

Certain cases stand out in my mind as exemplary of human beings' commitment to their pets. Peanuts Candelero the rat was one such case.

It was early in my internship. As usual, I had the night shift—the emergency shift, the one involving trauma and drama and oddball cases. Peanuts definitely fell into the last category.

He'd been named for his favorite food. He was three years old, with a life expectancy of maybe four years. That was in the best of all possible worlds, but that's where Peanuts was living. He'd been released from this same hospital only the day before, after having a large tumor removed from his groin. That operation cost more than some people would have spent on their dogs, but Peanuts's owners never hesitated.

Tonight, only two days post-op, he looked like a goner.

"He won't eat, and he just lies there," said the nine-year-old boy who called this creature a friend. His concern showed in his eyes; he was trying not to cry. His dad stood behind him, hands on the young man's shoulders.

"How long has he been like this?" I asked, cradling the rodent in one hand and gently going over him with the other. He was cold and dry and limp. His gums were pale. His long, hairless tail drooped lifelessly and his whiskers didn't twitch. I felt a rock-like mass in his abdomen. He barely flinched when I squeezed it. This was not good.

"Just a few hours. This morning he was fine. He was sitting on Timmy's lap eating peanuts. His favorite food."

"Any vomiting? Diarrhea?"

Two heads moved slowly back and forth. "He hasn't pooped at all!" said Timmy.

Bingo! The lights went on inside my head. "Were they salted peanuts?"

They were.

"I think he has an impaction." Rats possess two large pouches called ceca that branch off the sides of the intestine where the small intestine meets the large one. I remembered that from first-year anatomy class, where rodent anatomy had been something of an afterthought. Another species that has such an organ—though only one—is the horse. In horses, the cecum is prone to serious impaction, or filling with dried ingesta which forms a solid lump leading to pain, constipation, and further dehydration, along with all the sequelae to those developments. I was sure that's what I was feeling in Peanuts's belly, albeit on a smaller scale.

I tried to explain this to the Candeleros. "All that dry, salty food so soon after his operation must have been too hard for him to digest," I told them. "It balled up inside him and can't go anywhere. What I have to do is get it to break up and move out of there." Simplistic, maybe, but Peanuts didn't have a lot of time, and I lacked experience in explaining complicated physiological problems to pet owners. I said what mattered, and what I believed to be true: "He's got a chance."

The little guy's temperature was only 94 degrees, however, and his depression profound. "I'll need to admit him back into the hospital," I said cautiously. "He'll have to stay at least overnight in the incubator, and he needs fluids and maybe a stool softener. But I don't know if any of it will help. If he's still not passing stool by tomorrow, he may need surgery." I wondered if colic surgery on a rat was practical. I hoped I wouldn't have to find out.

Dad looked at son. "Well, we have to try," he said.

I prepared a cost estimate and presented it to them with some trepidation. After all, how much could one expect people to spend on a rat?

Mr. Candelero looked at the amount and sighed. "I sure wish he'd stop doing these things," he said fatalistically. He signed at the bottom.

Peanuts was already languishing in the incubator. I warmed some electrolyte solution and added a little glucose, then injected it into his abdomen, as I remembered one should do with "lab animals." I put him back in the incubator and went to see another case. An hour later I came back to find Peanuts alert and investigating his new surroundings.

I placed a small container of water in front of him and he drank. He circled the enclosure and drank again. During the night he consumed his body weight in water. He also chewed his way out of the incubator through plastic shields meant to allow caregivers to place their hands into the enclosure without disturbing the micro-environment. After that I moved him to a regular cage.

Peanuts taught me several things. One: Many medical concepts are transferable between species. Two: Rats have remarkable recuperative powers. And three: Never underestimate the power of the bond between a human and his pet.

I looked at Peanuts and saw a rodent, something that could be replaced for four or five dollars at the nearest pet store. He was also a medical challenge, and a good story to tell.

But Peanuts's owners had brought me a family member who was ill. They did not think of him in terms of his monetary value, or his life expectancy, or his social stature. He was simply their pet, and they had every right to expect me to treat him the same way I would a cat or dog.

Over the years I have treated a few rats, gerbils, rabbits, hamsters, ferrets, and two chinchillas. The owners' feelings toward their pets spanned the same spectrum I see in any group of pet owners. Not everyone who obtains a "free" kitten in the grocery store parking lot or adopts a puppy from the local shelter feels he or she has acquired a thing of value. Likewise, some owners of "pocket pets" seem to feel that we, as veterinarians, should charge them less because of the small size or short life expectancy of the animal. I can't change any of these attitudes, and I've learned to accept that.

But occasionally I let one of them change me.

The Patient Factor

Puddy's owner insisted the cat had not eaten in four weeks. Looking at the Siamese crouched on my table, I could believe it. Weighing in at around four pounds, she was so thin and dehydrated, her body so dry and stiff, she felt as though rigor mortis had already set in.

But that wasn't why Tiffany Smith had brought her twenty-one-year-old pet to see me.

"I think she's having trouble breathing," she said.

What an understatement. The cat held her neck carefully extended, mouth open, maximizing air flow. Her sides heaved with the effort. Even so, her blue gums testified to the futility of that effort. When I placed the bell of my stethoscope against her jutting ribs, I heard only an ominous silence.

Tiffany didn't look much older than the cat. She must have seen something in my face because she began crying. "Is she going to die? I've had this cat my whole life!"

"Tell you what," I said. "Have a seat out front and let me get some chest films and let's go from there." I studied her for a moment. "Or, if you'd prefer, you can wait in here."

"I can't come with her?" She was young enough to ask instead of demand.

"Not while we're taking X-rays." As gently as possible, I scooped up her pet and slipped out of the room.

The films revealed no surprises. Puddy's thorax was full of fluid. The lungs, which should have filled the chest cavity, were shrunken to a quarter their usual size. No wonder she wasn't getting enough air.

I placed the cat in our incubator and turned on the oxygen. I took the radiographs into the exam room, where Tiffany sat blot-

48

ting her eyes with a tissue. Tissues, unfortunately, are standard furnishings in a veterinary exam room.

"It's probably heart failure. Cardiomyopathy. But I can't tell for sure." I outlined a treatment plan, emphasizing the poor prognosis, both short- and long-term. Tiffany sniffled, her glazed eyes making me realize how little she was taking in.

We were both new at our roles. She'd grown up with this cat, had no pre-Puddy memories. Puddy had been spayed at the age of three, and hadn't seen a veterinarian since. Bringing her cat to me was one of her first responsible acts as an adult. Her goal had been getting here. Getting someone to take over. She had given no thought to what would happen after she arrived.

Moving trancelike, she came back to see the cat in her incubator. She went up front, signed the estimate and left a deposit using her parents' credit card. When she called fifteen minutes later to check on her cat, I knew she'd barely arrived home.

Puddy endured a series of carefully orchestrated procedures. First, we clipped and prepped her chest and drained the fluid. It was the first chest tap I'd ever done, and I read the appropriate section in two separate textbooks, then called a more experienced clinician before proceeding. It was surprisingly easy.

However, Puddy did not immediately breathe better. I left her in the incubator, breathing pure oxygen, and rationalized that her lungs needed a little time to recover. To re-expand.

After a while we got her out again and put in an IV catheter. I drew blood and urine and submitted them with the thoracic fluid to the lab.

Next, an electrocardiogram. I hooked her up to a slow drip of lactated Ringer's solution, trying to rehydrate her desiccated tissues. She refused an offer of baby food. Her body had been in "dying" mode for a long time. I couldn't expect her to change course so quickly. But she needed calories.

Lasix, ironically, was the first drug I gave her. I say "ironically" because it's a diuretic. It pulls fluid from tissue. Then Captopril, a vasodilator, to reduce the pressure on her heart. Then taurine, an amino acid only recently discovered by Dr. Paul Pion as a requirement in cats' diets, and not yet incorporated into most commercial cat foods. Aminophylline to help open the airways.

I spent the night staring into that incubator, hoping the cat would make it; waiting for the lab results; trying to force-feed baby food, give the poor creature some nutrients to fight back with. The following morning I might ultrasound her chest, confirm that I was dealing with dilatative cardiomyopathy. It's a disease we rarely see anymore in cats, thanks to taurine. But during my internship I dealt with three such cases.

How things have changed. I think about Puddy's case and how I might have managed her today. She'd have received oxygen via a tube glued into one nostril—such a simple concept but so slow to catch on. I'd have put another tube down the other nostril, and fed her with liquid diets designed for feeding that way. The lab results would have been available immediately, in-house. We have new drugs, chest tubes if needed. I could monitor her electrolytes and her blood gases, blood pressure and ECG, and fine-tune her treatment according to changes in any of these parameters.

None of which are likely to have made a bit of difference to Puddy.

She stabilized. After three days in the hospital she grudgingly accepted clam juice, rich in taurine, and occasionally licked at a plate of gourmet cat food. I sent her home with pale pink gums and three kinds of pills. She was breathing much better and could walk across the room without falling over. If I placed my stethoscope against her chest I could hear her pounding heart—it sounded like my first car's engine the day before it quit for good, but at least it was beating.

I felt proud. I'd saved my patient.

I called the next day. Tiffany was hanging in there. She wanted to do everything she could for Puddy, but the cat hated those pills. It was getting harder to make her swallow them. How long would she have to do this?

For the cat's entire life.

The next day Tiffany told me she wasn't going to give her cat any more pills. Her voice was clear and she sounded a little relieved to be telling me. "I've had her my whole life," she said. "And she's always been on my lap, or next to me when I was home. She used to sleep with me. Now she runs away when she sees me coming. She thinks I'm going to give her a pill. I know she's going to die soon, and it might take longer if I keep making her take the medicine. But she hates me! I don't want her to hate me. I'm not giving her any more pills."

I opened my mouth to protest, but I couldn't think of a single argument that made sense.

I've thought about that conversation a lot over the years. It was the first time I'd really been confronted with an animal who chose not to participate in its own survival. Perhaps if Tiffany had brought her in sooner, things would have been different. Or maybe not.

I sometimes believe that certain animals have simply accepted their own impending deaths and want nothing to do with our intervention. But the cases that gave me this feeling were inevitably those that had progressed to a near-death situation before I got them. I wonder if there isn't a point at which things have simply gone too far, and the ego—or whatever part of an animal's brain that is concerned with survival—just gives up.

These pets humble me time after time. I can't pick them out when they arrive. I've treated animals I thought were beyond saving, only to have them recover with a vengeance once the primary disease process was controlled. Others, who had no discernible reason to die, have crashed and burned while I looked on helplessly. It's an intangible factor—a will to live or die—that I cannot explain to a distraught owner.

Our patients are as individual as we are.

In several cases, I have known it was possible to keep an animal alive indefinitely. I have even done it, for days at a time. Yet once the animal gives up, nothing we do will change its mind.

It was an important lesson. I never heard from Tiffany again, but I'll always recall Puddy. I hope the end was easy for both of them.

Careful
What You Wish For

It was the job of my dreams: an equine hospital, with all the bells and whistles.

I'd arranged from the first to have the option of leaving the internship early if: (1) I found an equine job in the spring and (2) my classmate passed her state board exam that January.

She passed. I went interviewing. I was offered a job.

I moved to California's High Desert, expecting to spend my life there. My employer—I'll call him Boss—had received over a hundred resumes for the position. His associate was leaving April first, and he needed someone who could get in the truck and go, with nothing but a Thomas guide and the radio for directions. Someone who knew horses, knew medicine, but didn't have "unrealistic" salary expectations—though he paid better than most. I arrived giddy with excitement and ready to work.

Nine months later I was an irritable, defensive wreck. Despite working twelve-hour days and every other weekend, not one thing I'd done was quite right. If a client questioned something I'd said, Boss immediately promised he'd talk to me about it—but he never asked for my version of what happened. On a slow day I wasn't working hard enough, but if I brought in a huge pile of receipts I was overcharging his clients and they were sure to go elsewhere. More than once we sat down and agreed on a new hospital policy, only to have him change his mind without telling me. But when I didn't know his policy, there'd be hell to pay.

He rarely raised his voice. The only time he swore at me was the day I told him I was leaving. Usually he'd sort of wince and gaze at me with an air of disappointment that made me wonder why he tolerated me at all. The more this happened, the more real mistakes I made. Going to work became an ordeal. It was much later that I realized my combination of big-name references and female gender had doomed me from the start. Boss could not handle competent women.

I'd planned to give him ninety days to hire a replacement, but he screamed at me: *"You're an ass!"* and ordered me to leave his clinic. I was so relieved I didn't even mind being suddenly unemployed.

Such are the jobs of our dreams.

I had already gotten out the journals and begun the familiar task of sorting through openings. I no longer had the energy or the optimism for a long search, nor could I finance another cross-country move. Besides, I liked living in California.

That meant equine work was behind me. At that moment, I didn't really mind. I'd enjoyed my internship, especially the emergency work. The idea of working without a supervisor breathing down my neck held a certain appeal. So I searched for emergency clinic positions. Several were open, mostly in the Los Angeles area—not a place I wanted to live. Palm Springs was the closest one outside the city.

Anticipating this very situation, I had called the Palm Springs clinic the day before I left my job. The clinic opened at five. I called again soon after, and spoke again to the clinic director, Susan Klages.

"I'm available a little sooner than I expected," I told her.

"Do you want to come down for an interview later this week?"

I would have come that night. "Sure."

"How about Thursday at noon?"

I didn't have to check my calendar. "Okay."

"Here's my home phone number. When you get to town, stop and call me and I'll give you directions to the clinic. I'll meet you there and we can have lunch."

"Sounds good to me."

I dusted off a navy blue suit I'd bought for my original interviews following graduation, before figuring out that equine vets expected you to show your stuff. The suit hung loosely—I'd lost weight in the time I'd been in California. I found an old pair of panty hose with no visible runs. I left early, since I'd never been to Palm Springs and wasn't sure how long it would take.

By the time I arrived I was starving. I called the number she'd given me and was greeted by an obviously sleepy voice. Apparently the night before had been a busy one. Nevertheless, she gave me directions and said she'd be right down.

She arrived wearing sweatpants and a plaid work shirt. A cigarette dangled from her lips as if it lived there. She showed me around the clinic. The building was new; until a month ago the Animal Emergency Clinic of the Desert had been located across the street in the Animal Samaritans building, a low-cost spay/neuter clinic. Upheavals in that organization's operations had resulted in the need for a separate facility.

A lack of equipment gave the emergency clinic a roomy feel. There was plenty of work space, the floor plan reasonably efficient. It boasted a minimal laboratory, a small, WWII-vintage X-ray machine, and open tanks of chemicals for laborious hand development of the films.

I met the clinic cats: Texas, a twelve-year-old Maine coon rip-off whom Sue had saved to be a blood donor when his owners, traveling through in their motor home, could not delay their trip for their cat's medical treatment, and Red, a long-haired red tabby, who she had found tied to a post outside one morning. He'd been allowed to stay by virtue of the fact that Tex put up with him.

We sat in the small office-cum-lounge behind the front desk. A cast-off dining room table, a few cheap chairs and a disreputable futon were arranged to accommodate the office manager's desk. I picked one of the chairs, Sue another. Tex jumped into my lap and settled down to stay. Sue lit up a cigarette. We talked. My stomach growled and I shifted uncomfortably in the unaccustomed panty hose. We discussed scheduling and she gave me a brief history of the clinic.

Finally, she asked, "You want to try this weekend?"

"The whole thing?" That was one of the things we'd talked about—a week-on, week-off schedule. She naturally wanted to see if I could handle the long weekends. Saturday noon until Monday morning at eight o'clock, to be precise. Forty-four hours straight. "Sure," I said, actually looking forward to it.

We shook hands and she left. Nothing was said about lunch.

I stopped at Carl's Jr. on my way home. I cruised Palm Canyon, and Highway 111, but did not spend much time in the resort. The mountain scenery was great, but I wasn't really into glitter.

I never went on another interview. I worked every weekend that month, and in February moved into a small house on five acres in Morongo Valley, still high desert but only half an hour from the clinic. Della had plenty of space, and went to work with me every day. I could hike mountains from my back door, never needing to get in my car. It was a healing place to live. A good place to work. For a year I was content to remain an associate veterinarian and nothing more.

The support staff at the time I joined AEC was sparse but skilled. MJ Hegarty, a young mother of three, doubled as weeknight technician and office manager. Sharon Conkle, who had been a veterinary technician since long before I'd contemplated vet school, lived an hour away but liked the challenge of emergency work. Gayle Nelson, who had weekends and graveyard shifts, was a single mother struggling to raise her teenaged daughter on the meager pay provided. She left within a few months for a much better position with Palm Springs Animal Control, where she remains to this day. There were a few others, part-time weekend help, none of whom stayed long.

It wasn't fancy, but it was a beginning.

A Misdiagnosis

It is the wont of veterinary students to listen to stories told by practitioners of their early days in practice. We listen that we may learn, may know what to expect, even though we have worked as kennel attendants or technicians in the past.

I recall being astonished by tales of first jobs—new graduates hired on by tired vets who gave them a quick tour, then took off for their first vacations in years. Even the interns at the university laughingly told of being thrown to the wolves their first months on duty.

And then it happened to my class. I had a brand new diploma that magically declared me Doctor, but somehow I felt like the same scared kid who couldn't name the Greater Epiploic Artery in Rounds. Suddenly there I was in an examination room, facing a client with my brain full of knowledge but with little sense of the relative importance of each fact.

I had other interns to compare notes with, and it was helpful to know we all felt it. With time, we would discover our strengths and weaknesses—but those weaknesses would become apparent only through mistakes. Those mistakes would be made on animals belonging to clients who trusted us. This realization made us slow. We stayed up late reading, talked endlessly about the minute details of our cases, used one another's progress to gauge our own. There was so much to know, and it was dismaying to realize we could not retain everything. Some days I felt I knew nothing at all, as if the place where all that information had been stored was inexplicably cut out of my brain.

The most glaring hole in my education was surgery. Unlike MDs, the family vet is expected to be able to treat every case that comes through the doors. People burn out trying to live up to these expectations. In the course of a day we must be Internist, Radiologist, Dentist, Dermatologist, Cardiologist . . . and Surgeon. All these skills may be faked, with the help of texts, photos, and verbal consultations, except for surgery.

Surgical skills must be developed through practice. It is a talent learned as much by the hands and eyes as the mind. The procedures are described and illustrated, but one cannot learn the feel of living organs without handling them. I'd had good teachers, knew the concepts of sterile technique, minimizing tissue trauma, maximizing visibility, maintaining body temperature. But my hands were clumsy with a scalpel, slow and awkward and lacking in confidence when handling instruments, and my eyes were unreliable in assessing tissue viability.

Not coincidentally, it is the operating room that a responsible employer is least willing to consign to the new graduate. For it is here that a relatively small mistake is most likely to have catastrophic consequences.

At the time I was hired by the Animal Emergency Clinic of the Desert, I had performed very little real surgery. In veterinary school, during Didactic block, we students performed a series of procedures on castaway dogs: the routine spay, a fracture repair, these were things we expected to encounter regularly in practice. We practiced an intestinal anastomosis—removing a section of intestine and sewing the newly created ends together. We even opened the thoracic cavity to remove a lung lobe, a procedure I have yet to find a use for in practice. Each of us performed half these procedures, and assisted in the other half.

Later, in Surgery Rotation, students were allowed to perform elective procedures—spays, neuters, cat de-claws—under supervision, and only after first assisting while an intern did one. Depending on the caseload, we might do as many as two with our own hands. I was once given the privilege of removing a bone pin after a cat's leg had healed. It amounted to a half-inch skin incision and tugging the metal rod out with an instrument resembling a pair of pliers—though much more expensive, of course. Then stitching up the wound. I swelled with the responsibility of the task.

For more elaborate procedures, however, we stood as scrubbed observers, occasionally permitted to hand over an instrument, retract tissues so the surgeon could see what he was doing, or hold the suction tip to remove fluids pumped in by a resident. And of course, we cut the sutures while the surgeon sewed. This did not prepare us for practice.

My internship, in a private veterinary practice, was only a small step above this. Again relegated to retracting and cutting sutures, my only real experience came at night. Just as in the stories I'd heard, there I would find myself, the only doctor on duty, often with a technician who was openly contemptuous of my untested skills, and therefore a less than ideal assistant. I learned to sew up lacerations, remove fishhooks from puppy lips, open and drain cat-fight abscesses, extract foxtails from ears and under the skin between toes. But if "real" surgery was needed, the real surgeon was called in.

Working on horses after my internship did not afford me more surgical experience. But it did teach me to think on my feet, far from the clinic, with no other DVM to back me up and no handy book to consult. This was extremely useful later on.

During my first weekend as an aspiring emergency clinician, a small dog came in with a badly damaged eye. It was clear nothing could return the ruptured globe to function, so it had to be removed. I had performed exactly one enucleation before, under the auspices of Dr. Dennis Hacker, an ophthalmologist, during my internship. I remembered two things: It's important to remove all the tear-producing glands in order to prevent cysts from forming later, and the ophthalmic artery bleeds like a geyser.

The dog's owner, relieved not to have to look at the awful thing anymore, turned her pet over to me with the sort of trust that scared me worse. As I prepared the little dog for surgery, the president of the emergency clinic's board of directors, Dr. Doug Kunz, stopped by to meet me. I understood he was gaining an impression of my suitability for the position. (If I'd asked, he probably would have performed the operation for me. And I most likely would not have been hired.) He was polite and cheerful, but he showed no sign of leaving anytime soon.

Quaking inside, I went forward with the surgery while he watched. I clipped the hair around the bulging mess and scrubbed the area with surgical soap. I pulled on sterile gloves and cut a small round hole in a paper drape to keep my field as clean as possible.

Mounting a blade on a scalpel, I attempted my initial incision. The soft tissue sunk in, uncut. Even a sharp blade needed to push against something. I needed a firm backing that would slip beneath the eyelid and give counterpressure to the scalpel. Thinking furiously, I glanced at the instruments in my hands. The tweezerlike thumb forceps were broad and flat at the base, a good impromptu support. I flipped it around—it worked!

Almost involuntarily, I glanced at Dr. Kunz. He watched with something like amusement on his face. Perhaps he knew exactly what I was going through, or maybe I had him convinced this was a piece of cake. He didn't say. But he did leave halfway through the operation. And it only took me forty-five minutes, about twice what it takes me today. And two weeks later, when I took the sutures out, the scar was straight and even, and the skin had healed perfectly. I'd proved myself to the board.

More important, I'd proved myself to myself.

The enucleation was straightforward enough—hardly invasive, with minimal potential for serious complications. After the first one, I did almost one a month for as long as I worked there. It became routine.

Other procedures, however, were more intimidating. Eventually, I knew, I would have to tackle the worst sorts of emergency procedures. Every new vet's worst fears—diaphragmatic hernias and gastric dilatation-volvulus syndromes and intestinal perforations—tend to present themselves at night and on weekends. And, inevitably, they came.

The first time I was presented with a diaphragmatic hernia—a perforation in the flat muscle separating the chest from the abdominal cavity, through which the abdominal contents often slide, cutting off their own circulation and interfering with breathing—I was able to call in a local vet with a reputation as an excellent surgeon. He performed the procedure and the dog recovered well.

The second one was a kitten. It was in bad shape when it arrived, but its owner wanted to do everything possible to save it. I placed the kitten in our incubator, with oxygen running full-force, and tried without success to reach someone I thought could pull it through. The kitten couldn't wait. I was going to have to attempt to repair it myself. We got it out of the incubator to anesthetize it, and it died on the spot. The minor stress of handling killed it. There was no way this kitten would have survived the kind of operation it needed. I admit to feeling slightly relieved, though vastly disappointed.

The third one was a surprise.

One night, during the spring of my second year at the Emergency Clinic, a young shar-pei came in after being missing for two days. "ADR" was written on the chart: tongue-in-cheek shorthand for "Ain't Doing Right"—a very common complaint that means nothing, or might mean anything at all.

Delilah was a bitch, in both senses of the word. She was unspayed and bleeding from the vulva, but not swollen. The owner reported that she had been in heat about two months earlier. She had a moderate fever of 104 degrees. I muzzled her and performed my examination: aside from the fever, Delilah appeared listless and irritable—or that may just have been her personality. She was mildly dehydrated and tender in the abdomen—at least I assumed so, because she tried even harder to bite me when I gently attempted palpation. Her breathing was rapid and shallow, not a pant exactly, but not really normal. I attributed that to the muzzle.

Delilah's owner was an elegant woman, tall and black and with the bearing of an actress. Her every move was efficient. Next to her I felt clumsy and inept. I wanted to impress this person. I wanted to be confident and correct, someone she would approve of.

With all the confidence I could muster, I said, "Delilah has a uterine infection called a pyometra." Not "I need to run some diagnostic tests, then we'll see." Not even "I think she has pyometra." I said, "The only treatment is surgery to remove the infected organ." Pyometra was simple. I knew how to handle pyometra. The history was right: in heat eight weeks ago, the vaginal drainage, and the fever. But even then I was thinking the discharge didn't look quite right.

Delilah's owner accepted everything I told her. "I kept meaning to get her fixed," she said ruefully, when she saw the cost estimate. We joked that it would have been cheaper a few weeks ago, and she left.

So sure was I of my diagnosis that I did not x-ray the dog's abdomen, nor did I perform any lab work to confirm an elevated white blood cell count. In the case of a pyometra where the cervix is open and the pus can drain out, these tests are often normal, and that's what I assumed was going on here. Our lab and X-ray equipment of the day left much to be desired, and under the circumstances these tests seemed more trouble than they were worth. Had I done them, and had the results been normal, it would not have changed my diagnosis.

However, it would have told me more about her other organs. As it turned out, that information could have made a huge difference.

We prepared her for major surgery: intravenous fluids and antibiotics, followed by light anesthesia induction and gas maintenance. I made my incision fairly low on the abdomen, to access the uterus. I was puzzled by the minimal inflammation there, but reasoned that we'd caught the condition early and, since the cervix was open, the uterus had not filled with pus the way others in my experience had done. I proceeded with the hysterectomy and finished in record time, feeling a little uneasy now but still convinced my diagnosis was correct.

The uterus gone, I began closing the incision. And heard, for the first time, the telltale hiss of air moving. Air in a place where it should not be moving.

"Oh, shit," I said.

Sharon, the veterinary technician, met my eyes, hers wide with alarm. "She was gone two days. Think she got hit by a car?"

Of course she had. *Click,* the pieces suddenly fell into place. Her uterus wasn't infected, she was in heat. Either she hadn't been in heat at all two months earlier, or the short cycle was an aberration—not surprising in a breed known for its aberrations. She'd come in heat, and escaped to find a male. I pictured her, injured by a car, holed up under a bush somewhere, trying to catch her breath and waiting for the pain to abate enough that she could walk home.

The hole in her diaphragm was tiny. No organs had passed through it. It would not have shown up on X-rays. She would not have gone to surgery at all, had I not misread the history and symptoms. Maybe that was a good thing. Untreated, this hole could easily enlarge with time, causing chronic herniation, vague long-term symptoms, and possibly death or a much more complicated operation in the distant future.

So I reasoned. I immediately enlarged my incision and probed with my fingers for the defect. Sharon started "bagging" the dog—inflating her lungs, since she couldn't breathe now—while I stitched. It was very easy, as these things go, and I had the rip repaired in twenty minutes—very fast for me in those days.

It was good that Delilah's diaphragm was now repaired. It was good that she was spayed.

It was bad that I hadn't x-rayed her chest, because the kind of trauma that causes a diaphragmatic hernia makes lungs bleed. It makes them leak.

Today I would automatically place a chest tube after a procedure like this. At the time not only had I never placed a chest tube, but as far as I knew, neither had any vet in the entire Coachella Valley. Chest tubes were considered extreme. They require a lot of maintenance, and given Delilah's disposition, high maintenance was not a good idea.

However, her breathing never improved. She awoke from the anesthetic as irritable and snappy as ever. I called her owner and explained what had happened. She handled the news calmly as I would have expected. Like me, she thought it was remarkably lucky we had gone in and discovered the hernia.

The next morning Delilah was transferred to her regular vet. Her condition had not changed overnight. During that day, nothing was done to help her. The staff was afraid of her. She lay in her kennel breathing rapidly and shallowly, and that night they sent her back to the emergency clinic.

I wasn't working that night. Another local veterinarian, Ann Blakely, was filling in, giving me a welcome night off. I stopped in anyway, and there was Delilah. She'd been put back on her drip, she'd had an antibiotic injection, and that was it. She was still breathing the same way. She bared her teeth and growled if I moved to touch her. I wished we had a practical way to administer oxygen to her. I wished Ann would do a chest X-ray, but I could see why she and the staff were reluctant to handle the dog to that extent.

"What do you think about this one?" I asked Dr. Blakely.

She said, "I've been leaving it alone. It's not really my case."

"Think she needs a chest tap?"

She shrugged. I later learned that, in fifteen years of practice, Ann Blakely had never performed a chest tap. However, I had barely three years' experience, one of those with horses. I deferred to her judgment.

Delilah died that night. I don't know whether my opening her up and repairing her diaphragm contributed to her death. Surgical stress can be tremendous. I suspect her willingness to bite did contribute, because it made her tough to work with, and there's no real solution to that problem when it occurs. Or maybe she was going to die no matter what we did. But I honestly believe that, had I been less afraid of that thoracic cavity, more willing to x-ray, tap, evacuate, to face the owner and tell her there were things I didn't know, tests she would have to pay for to give us the information we needed, that Delilah might have been saved. It would require a confidence I then lacked, and a willingness to approach the owner with new fees. Because, though I never got a chance to prove it, I'm convinced now that Delilah died because her lungs were collapsed by blood and air.

Delilah was a case that changed how I approach other cases. Part of the problem was my lack of experience, and part of it was the lack of available equipment. But the real reason Delilah died nine years ago and, I believe, would not have died today, is my change of attitude that has occurred in that small amount of time. When I graduated from vet school the only practical way to administer oxygen to a pet was by placing that animal in an oxygen cage. They were noisy, isolated, terrifying units, they were very expensive and they took up a lot of space. We did not have one to accommodate even a medium-sized dog. Even at school, no one ever suggested we place a tube into a dog's nostril to administer oxygen. I knew it was being done elsewhere, but I'd never seen it in practice. Shortly after Delilah's death I purchased a used oxygen concentrator—a device often used for humans in the home. It runs on electricity and pulls oxygen out of the air, concentrates it and pumps it through saline for humidity, then shoots it down any length of tubing to the animal (or human) at the other end. The tubing fit the inexpensive feeding tubes, which could be comfortably inserted into a canine or feline nostril. This arrangement is still used routinely at the emergency clinic, and I have no doubt lives have been saved as a result. But at the time Delilah was in the hospital, this was not available.

Delilah also made me more aggressive with diagnostics. I'm quicker to recommend X-rays and blood work, both noninvasive tests that can result in a lot of information. And, perversely, she led me to be more willing to use surgery as a diagnostic tool. I would not have suspected that hernia had I not seen it, thrust a finger through it. I'll never forget that sound: air moving through a small, wet space. I'll always remember the thrill I felt when that hole was sealed.

Today I would handle a Delilah differently. But I'll never know if it would have mattered.

Moving Up

I joined AEC in January of 1989, officially accepting the full-time associate position on February 1. It was a frightening step—my entire education had, I thought, been aimed at a very different sort of practice. With horse owners I felt confident, even cocky—I had something in common with each, and frankly, equine medicine involved little in the way of variety. Now, despite my internship and the good reviews I'd received from my teachers in small animal clinics, I felt like an imposter.

People came, bringing their sick pets, and actually listened to—and followed!—my advice. All the while a voice in the back of my head was whispering, *"What are you doing? What made you think you could pull this off?"* If anyone else heard the voice, they never let on.

I believed the staff thought me incompetent—I now understand this came from my own fear that I was in over my head. One partial internship a year earlier did not qualify me to be the only veterinarian on call for an hour or more in any direction. What's more, my time at the equine hospital had left me jumpy and defensive—whenever my employer there had said, "We need to talk," it meant, "You screwed up again, and I want to tell you about it." Those words triggered tension and apprehension. It was a long time before I realized all those "transgressions" at my previous job had nothing to do with my ability to practice medicine.

So it was like starting over, but with baggage. First I needed to mourn my image of myself as a horse doctor. Getting into and then through vet school was the first time I'd set a major goal and achieved it. For all those years I'd had a pretty realistic idea what to expect—as long as I could work on horses. Had it really taken less than a year of actually doing it to drive that out of me?

A third major move in three years landed me in a small house on five acres in Morongo Valley, about half an hour from the clinic. Della loved it, and loved going to work with me. She accepted the change with her usual complacency.

At first, I knew no one outside work, could not afford to travel. My schedule gave me alternating weeks off—time I spent closeted with books. I've always been an ardent reader of fiction. I never got the television habit. I read and read and read. I'd pick up a veterinary journal, read half an article, go back to the latest Dick Francis novel. It was a way of escaping my own life, a vacation from goal-setting.

I missed the regimented predictability and built-in social life in school. Considered going back—law school? Medical school? A residency perhaps—I'd once hoped to be a surgeon.

Yet more poverty. Another big commitment. I postponed the necessary phone calls, the ones that would result in the arrival in my mailbox of letters and brochures and application forms. Deadlines came and went.

This, my third year out of school, I was paid a salary of $32,000. That sounded like a lot when the offer was made—it represented an increase from what I took home from the equine hospital. But after taxes it barely covered rent, student loan payments, installments on my 1985 Nissan pickup—hardly a luxury vehicle—car insurance and basic necessities, with enough for an occasional dinner out at Sizzler or Baker's Square.

I did squeeze out fifteen dollars a month for a membership in a gym in nearby Yucca Valley. Small-animal practice was sedentary work!

I languished. Instead of working to meet the challenge presented by my new job, I was learning to fake it. No wonder I felt like a fraud when I walked into an exam room—I was acting like one! I had moved to the desert thinking this would be another in a string of temporary jobs. Before and after school, that's how I had lived. Why should I expect my new life to be different?

Two things happened to subtly alter my way of thinking.

The first was meeting a woman who would become the closest adult friend I'd ever known. She's an attorney named Joan Baumgarten, and I met her in the law library while researching my rights regarding my former landlord from equine practice days. The property management company had refused to return my security deposit, citing bogus damages and losses. I was determined to get my money back, and eventually won a settlement in small-claims court. Joan was in the library that day. We chatted for hours and went to dinner, the first of many over the years. I had not recognized a fundamental loneliness in myself; making a friend helped.

The second event was the departure from the emergency clinic of the only director it had known in its brief existence. Sue Klages announced in October her intention to leave on the first of the year, to buy into Eldorado Animal Hospital in Palm Desert. A vacuum was thus created between myself and the board of directors, some of whom I had never met.

I never got to know Sue well. We worked opposite shifts; she had a child and a mate and a life apart from the clinic. We had nothing in common; we would never quite be friends. However, I respected her work and the enormous, even awe-inspiring effort involved in seeing the new building constructed and moving the practice into it. That would be her legacy, then. After almost ten years of practice, she was making the break into ownership.

Having known me only in my capacity as a somewhat apathetic associate, Sue reasonably recommended against promoting me to fill her position. I, too, assumed I was not qualified to manage. A search ensued. A smattering of unenthused applicants drifted through the clinic. I was not invited to participate in the selection process, but it was interesting to observe. I began to see that I was not the only person to struggle toward a goal only to see the goal evaporate like a mirage when reached. As the saying goes, life was happening despite the best-laid plans.

This revelation energized me. Of the applicants I'd met, none was particularly qualified to run our emergency clinic. Months passed, Sue trying to manage from a distance, me working extra shifts to pick up the slack. Summer loomed. With a "what have I got to lose?" attitude, I updated my resume and mailed a copy to each board member.

I was too late.

At my first board meeting I got the news. The board members—each of whom owned a practice in the area, referred emergency cases to me, and had a different opinion of what the emergency clinic should be—were all present: Bob Maahs, independently wealthy and considering retirement; Vicki Robertson, who perhaps regretted her recent purchase of one of the oldest practices in Palm Springs upon the death of its founder; Doug Kunz, an easy-going father figure always ready with advice or encouragement; Sam Jackson, whose showplace hospital nestled at the foot of a mountain in Rancho Mirage served as a local landmark; and Bob Cockcroft, an eccentric giant, standing nearly seven feet tall and practicing only on cats.

"We've hired a new director," Doug told me. He looked at Sam. No one was meeting my eyes.

Sam said, "His name is Jim Baker. He just sold his practice in New Mexico. I offered him the job while I was at Western States" (a huge veterinary convention held annually in Las Vegas).

I wasn't sure how to react to this news. Who was this person who would be my new boss, who had been hired without even visiting the clinic he proposed to manage? Well, I had no real attachments. There were other jobs if it didn't work out. The thought made me tired.

"He'll only be at the clinic for six months to a year," Sam went on. "After that, he'll come to work for me full-time."

Six months. Maybe a year. "And then?" I asked.

Board members exchanged glances. They had talked about this ahead of time. "Yours is the best resume we've received," Vicki said. "Consider this a training period."

Yes! I was in! Or would be, eventually.

Jim, in fact, never really managed the Animal Emergency Clinic of the Desert. From the beginning he worked part-time at the practice Sam Jackson then owned half of, Desert View Animal Hospital. He would soon move into a full-time position there, leaving night work behind him. That was clearly his main focus, and he made no pretense otherwise.

Tentatively, almost in self-defense, I took on jobs Sue had performed before. MJ had left the previous autumn and had never been successfully replaced, so office manager tasks also fell to the director. These included payroll, a definite priority, and basic accounting. She'd shown Jim most of what was involved and had made notes on pertinent topics, notes that I found in drawers and files and "in" boxes.

The need for new staff galvanized me. The void left when MJ quit for a daytime job had never been filled. Another technician announced her plan to follow Sue to her new practice. Within days we would be critically short-staffed. Jim was still a bit dazed after the move from New Mexico and starting two new jobs simultaneously. He showed no sign of dealing with the impending crisis.

By lucky coincidence, we'd received a letter from a young undergraduate student named Rebecca Kemp, who lived in Cherry Valley, nearly an hour away. She hoped to attend veterinary school one day, and needed job experience. Her brother lived in Palm Springs, making the Coachella Valley convenient for her. I called her in for an interview.

Rebecca joined the staff of AEC at age nineteen. She has left for various academic pursuits, but as of this writing, seven years later, still fills in.

Hiring Rebecca was the first step I took toward taking up the reins of management. The job, which had seemed impossibly complicated from my previous observation point, proved reachable. The trick, I learned, was staying on top of it. I used the months that Jim Baker was officially at the helm to formulate a plan. The staff needed better pay, and we desperately needed better equipment. However, the money had to come from somewhere. That meant not only raising our fees, and sticking with them, but utilizing the diagnostics we already had. Most of all, it meant honing my own skills so that certain cases did not intimidate me.

Suddenly I had a new goal.

Was That
A Bullet?

Today I look forward to performing surgery. I enjoy exploring an abdomen, not sure what I'll find. There have been times when I got started on something, got to the point of no return, and realized I was in over my head. But patience and persistence always paid off, and almost all the animals I operated on did well in the end, if they were capable of doing well.

The criteria I used in deciding whether to go forward were simple: If I could refer the case to a more qualified surgeon, I did so. The board-certified scalpels were two hours away, however, and many could not wait that long. In those cases, I made a diligent effort to call in a more experienced veterinarian. If that failed, I felt I had no choice but to give it my best shot. Once I'd done one successfully, I felt I could handle the next without seeking help. It turned out to be a good system.

Pyometras came and went, cesarean sections and huge ulcerated tumors that had grown for months became emergencies when they started to bleed. Tedious procedures, but good practice.

One case stands out as completely altering my confidence in my own abilities. I'd been at the emergency clinic for about two years.

The dog's name was, ironically, Bullet. He was a huge mutt, a 110-pound mix of shepherd, mastiff, retriever, and who-knew, graceful and square-bodied, covered with a sleek layer of russet-and-black hair. He was two years old. He was not neutered, and that may have been his downfall.

It was Christmas Day, a Friday, which meant a four-day holiday weekend. I'd been on duty since noon on Thursday. Weekends like this one are either frantically busy or agonizingly slow. This one was busy.

Bullet lived with his owner over an hour from the clinic, at Salton Sea. The Salton Sea is a vast salt lake east of Palm Springs, the result of a burst pipeline spilling Colorado River water into the desert for two years, early in the century. It is not beautiful. There is no river flowing in or out, so the water is stagnant. It smells, and is murky on its best days. But it is the only recreational body of water anywhere nearby, and surrounding land is inexpensive. So a permanent population has grown on the lakefront: earthy, practical people for the most part. People who are glad the clinic is open when it's open, and do not complain about the long drive. They are used to driving.

Bullet walked in. He took short, careful steps, and even wagged his tail a little when I rubbed his ears. He had a hole the size of my little finger on the left side of his abdomen, and another on his right. His belly wall was rigid, and I did not try probing the puncture wounds.

Bullet had left his yard that morning, as usual, but had not returned. When his owner, Jim Walden, called him, he came hobbling down the road using much the same gait as he did to enter the clinic. Jim knew a gunshot wound when he saw one. He got out the phone book and called us, threw his pet in the back of his pickup truck, and brought him down.

Hoping illogically that the bullet could have traveled through Bullet's body without tearing anything important, I carefully x-rayed his belly. The detail was awful, due to the extreme inflammation and the very little fat this dog had to begin with, so I couldn't follow his intestinal tract on the films. But one thing was clear: There was sand in his belly, and it was not arranged in the linear clumps I'd seen when dogs ate sand and it traveled through their intestines. It may have started in his gut, but it was now free in the abdomen.

Bullet needed an exploratory laparotomy—which means going in without knowing what to expect—because he needed his intestines repaired and he needed it done now. He already had peritonitis and if I didn't fix the gut and get that sand out of there, it would kill him. And even if he had the very best surgeon, the best facility available anywhere, it might kill him anyway.

I already knew there would be no help locally, because I'd asked everyone who might help when I first scheduled the weekend. I was it.

Doing my best to sound competent, I explained the situation to Jim Walden. A lot of people would have put their dogs to sleep under the circumstances, but then most dogs wouldn't have been standing there wagging their tails after being shot, walking home, and riding in the back of a pickup for an hour. Jim nodded, said he understood the risks, signed the estimate form, and asked when we'd do the operation. I said, "As soon as possible," and he left.

Fortunately I had my best tech on duty. We got Bullet started on fluids and antibiotics and painkillers. More emergencies came in, things I couldn't put off while I operated on Bullet. A couple of hours went by. Finally I got to the first lull all day, and realized this might be my only chance to do the operation.

With Sharon's help, I anesthetized Bullet and got him ready. We had switched to isoflurane anesthetic gas a few months earlier, for which I was profoundly grateful now. Iso is faster and safer than its counterparts.

"We're out of oxygen," Sharon said.

"What?" It simply couldn't be. We needed oxygen to operate the anesthesia machine, to carry the gas into Bullet's lungs.

"Not totally out. But it's in the red."

Not totally out. How long would the little bit last? How could we get so low on oxygen without someone noticing?

There was no time to wait for an emergency delivery. I couldn't stop now. We turned Bullet's flow rate down to about what I'd use on a cat. I felt like a pilot running out of fuel over uncharted territory. The pressure was on.

We got the dog into the OR and I scrubbed my hands while Sharon prepared the dog's belly. I was gowned and gloved in record time, the pack open and a scalpel in my hand. The dog's skin parted beneath my blade. Another incision—the muscle layer—and I was in.

There was blood, which I had not expected. Every organ, every tissue I encountered was the angry purple-red of peritonitis. "Well, at least it's not black," I muttered. The inflammation I was looking at required an active blood supply. This was a belly that would probably do okay, if only I could repair the source of the insult—before we ran out of oxygen.

The bullet that tore through Bullet's abdomen had ripped his intestine in three places. The margins were shredded. I would have to cut out the bad pieces and suture the new ends together. Fortunately, as long as only small pieces were taken, the gut handled this procedure well. If it was done correctly.

The only resection I had done was back in school, almost four years ago. But I'd scrubbed in on a lot of colic surgery in horses, and the procedure was straightforward enough. The two primary complications one had to be careful of were leakage at the site of anastomosis and scar formation, which could lead to a stricture or a kink, and future obstructions. Scar tissue tended to result from trauma—in this case not the trauma of the bullet passing through, but the micro-trauma of rough handling during surgery. It was important not only to be fast, but also to be gentle.

I got to work. First I suctioned the blood pooling in Bullet's abdomen, which made visibility much better. I washed the intestine with saline and determined where I would cut—removing the most damaged part while leaving as much as possible. I clamped above and below, and made my incisions. Sharon handed me the suture material and I began the tedious process of putting the pieces together. First one stitch at the base—the mesenteric side, where blood flowed in, being extra careful not to cut off the all-important circulation. Then another on the opposite, antimesenteric side, so it wouldn't lose its shape while I worked. Then a whole series of tiny sutures, one millimeter apart, each with its own knot. It took a long time, and when I tested it afterward, it leaked fluid. I found the leak and placed yet another suture. No leak now. If they all held, this site should heal.

No time to celebrate. I had more damage to repair. The other two tears were only several inches apart when the gut was straightened out, and the strip between them did not look good. I removed the whole thing, so there was only one set of ends to sew together. It was slightly harder to get to, but I'd had a little practice now and was beginning to think Bullet would be okay. The anastomosis went smoothly. And it didn't leak this time.

Sharon already had several bags of saline warmed up, and

now she poured one into the belly. I sloshed the saline around—literally holding the sides of the incision and rocking the dog—and suctioned it out. It came back bloody and with a lot of sand in it. We repeated the process again and again. Several bags later the fluid came back clear and the gritty feel to the organs was replaced by the slick-smooth surface I'd learned to associate with tissues that wanted to live. Miraculously, the vital organs were untouched, as was the colon. I could not find the source of all that blood—I decided it must have come from the severed intestines. It was time to close.

I had sealed the muscle layer and was halfway through the subcutis when the dog took a breath that didn't go anywhere.

"Sew fast," Sharon said calmly. "You're out of air."

She disconnected the machine, so Bullet could breathe room air while I finished. Sharon put the skin stapler within reach and I asked her to give the dog a large injection of narcotic. He didn't start moving until I was placing the last few staples.

"Talk about down to the wire!" she said as we lifted the dog onto the gurney.

Bullet is still one of the most remarkable patients I've ever had. He went home Monday morning, already eating the small meals we allowed him, and clearly wanting more.

Wednesday evening, Jim Walden called to tell us Bullet had gotten out again, and been gone overnight. Now he was back, but he'd been sleeping all day. Should he worry? He was understandably reluctant to bring the dog back, so we decided to let the dog sleep it off. Thursday night, Walden stopped by for some tranquilizers for Bullet. He'd already bought materials to repair his fence.

Bullet was neutered by his regular vet a couple of weeks later. The staples came out at the same time. By then the anastomoses would be healed, and any risk of leakage was over. I'd done some reading by then, and it seemed that scarring was unlikely.

I don't know whether neutering slowed him down or not. I never saw the dog again. At any rate, Bullet's case was a milestone in my career. He had tested not just my surgical skills, but my ability to manage a complicated trauma case. Saving Bullet meant managing shock, pain, peritonitis, and infection from the primary injury. Bullet was unusually tough, but he had a potentially fatal wound. His was one case where medical intervention truly made all the difference. Without a doubt, my team had saved his life.

It was as wonderful a Christmas gift as any I've ever received.

Swan Songs

Among our many repeat clients were a few of the local country clubs and hotels that keep parrots and swans and even flamingos for the enjoyment of their guests and residents. I had the privilege of treating a young swan for burned feet after she eschewed the large lake at one hotel, preferring instead to follow guests along the pavement looking for handouts. She spent a week at the clinic, and I understand she never did learn to stay off the hot sidewalks.

One Saturday an injured male flamingo was delivered to me for safekeeping, until the caretakers could contact their regular vet on Monday. Despite his being kept in Isolation, away from the stress-inducing activity of the main Treatment area, an occasional client spotted him. The site of that elegant wading bird huddled in a cage obviously designed for a dog generated a fair number of double-takes.

"Is that a flamingo?" was the invariable question.

"Yes, it is," I would answer.

"What happened to it?"

"He was attacked by a swan."

That generally ended the conversation. No one could think what to say after that.

But swans were victims as well as aggressors. One swan suffered one of the few incidents of overt and pointless cruelty I have witnessed in my career. It was a beautiful young male, one of two hand raised and donated to the City of Palm Desert by a resort faced with a surplus of swans. They were placed on a pond in a city park. They trusted humans; they had no reason to fear them.

An adolescent boy had been witnessed by several passersby

throwing stones at the swans. Later the same day this one was presented to the emergency clinic with every sign of a concussion.

He had a large bruise at the base of his skull. His head drooped, though he was still conscious by the time he reached me. He collapsed on his chest, his head lying sideways on the floor of the run. His efforts at controlling that long, once-graceful neck were to no avail.

Aghast, I offered a guarded prognosis and began treatment as I would any other animal with head trauma. As I spent more time with him, I learned he enjoyed having the base of his neck scratched. If I supported his head, he could stand. After several hours he took water. The second day he began to try for food. Gradually his strength and coordination returned. After three or four days he went home, apparently normal.

Within a week both swans were dead.

I will never understand what drives anyone to destroy a thing of beauty, a helpless creature, unable to even comprehend the idea of striking back. I have seen animals struck in anger, dropped or stepped on by children, ears and extremities nearly lost to rubber bands placed carelessly. Once I treated a dog whose spleen had ruptured when an angry owner kicked him across the room, and was immediately penitent. But outright cruelty is, fortunately, rare.

I understand they caught the boy. I hear he got off with probation.

"Every Bone
In His Body"

Of course he had to be named Lucky.

They arrived on a Saturday evening, one of my long week-ends—I worked the whole thing. The pup wasn't much more than two weeks old, his eyes barely open. He was brown and white, of uncertain ancestry, and very, very thin. His left hind leg was mangled.

"We found him at the dump," Mrs. Henneke said, breathing hard as if she'd just run all the way to the clinic.

"Under the tire." Mr. Henneke seemed ashamed. "We didn't see him. I just heard this sound."

"This awful cry," said his wife. "It was horrible!"

While they talked, I examined the pup. Scrawny and filthy and dehydrated, he was otherwise in pretty good shape. That leg was a problem, though, torn nearly off halfway down the femur—the thighbone. The lower limb was cold to the touch, indicating it had lost its blood supply. It would have to be amputated.

Now, we got a lot of stray animals brought in to the emergency clinic, and the outcome depended largely on the people who brought them in. The fact that he had been found at the dump, and wasn't old enough to possibly survive on his own, meant the odds of another owner coming forth to claim the pup were astronomically remote. If no one was willing to pay its bills, and most important, offer it a permanent home, the pup would have to be put to sleep. I broached the subject gently.

"Assuming this little guy pulls though, are you willing to adopt him?"

I still recall Mr. Henneke's exact words: "My dear young lady, we have just spent the last eighteen hours driving nine hundred miles from La Paz, Mexico, to get this little puppy some medical care. I *think* we're going to keep him!"

As the story unfolded, it turned out the dump these folks had found the puppy in was not a domestic dump. They had a summer home in La Paz, a Mexican resort, and had been taking their trash to the dump when they discovered the helpless puppy beneath the tire of their car. They had, naturally, taken the creature to a local veterinarian—one who was quite proud of his facility, which boasted one of the few X-ray machines in a Mexican vet clinic. I suspect he did not get many opportunities to use it. They had brought the X-rays with them, and produced them now.

I put them up on the viewer.

"He said he'd broken every bone in his body," said Mrs. Henneke. "He told us to put him to sleep."

The films, though correctly exposed and developed, were appalling. Bare human hands held puppy feet in a twisted position not even reminiscent of anything I was used to. The actual fracture was obscured by skeletal fingers. However, the tiny puppy's bones were mostly cartilage, which does not show up on radiographs. There were a lot of gaps in the skeleton as a result. Two growth plates for each bone, in fact, for every bone in the little pup's body.

Trying hard not to laugh out loud, I pointed out what the well-meaning vet had seen, and explained what it meant. "It's perfectly normal. The only real problem is this leg."

They were relieved, but not terribly surprised.

I wanted to keep the puppy overnight, hydrate him, feed him, and start him on antibiotics prior to amputating the limb the following morning. The Hennekes were adamant that they would not leave him at the clinic. I never found out why they felt that way, but in the end I had to acquiesce. It was, after all, their dog, and I could do nothing without their permission. So I gave him an antibiotic injection and subcutaneous fluids, and bandaged the leg as best I could. I sent him home with a nurser and some formula. They would keep him at home and return the next morning for surgery.

I half-expected them not to show up. The prospect of anesthetizing a puppy that young for major surgery was something I looked forward to with a mixture of anticipation and dread. It was a familiar mix, the combined professional challenge and the knowledge that if something went wrong, I'd always blame myself.

They arrived, somewhat less harried than on the previous evening. The pup was more active, with a full stomach and bright, pink gums for a change.

And the leg was seriously starting to smell.

He was so tiny we could not get an endotracheal tube into his airway. I performed the entire amputation with a mask over Lucky's snout, delivering a mixture of isoflurane gas, the safe-but-expensive anesthetic we'd recently upgraded to, and oxygen.

Wanting to keep surgery time to a minimum, I simply removed the part of the leg that was already dead, trimmed the stump until bleeding indicated healthy tissue, and chipped the sharp points off the bone before sewing tissue over its end. I knew he would probably require another operation later, preferably not for a few weeks, and made sure the Hennekes knew this. He came out of the procedure lively and hungry.

I didn't see him for follow-up, but his regular vet updated me periodically. Lucky did indeed require another operation, to cut the bone back a little, because there was not enough muscle to cover it and it kept pushing through.

Years later, I had all but forgotten the incident. I was treating a cat for an abscess, and had to keep it for a few hours until it recovered from anesthesia. When its owners returned to pick it up, they brought along a three-legged dog named Lucky. He looked like a cross between a dachshund and a Chihuahua, unremarkable in appearance except for a twist in his body to keep his weight centered over his single hind leg. His face wore a cheerful grin and his tail wagged nonstop.

"Do you remember a little puppy from Mexico?" they asked.

"This is him?" I was thrilled to see him again, though of course the dog's affection was generic; he didn't remember me but he was glad to see everyone.

"I guess being run over by your car in that dump was the best thing that ever happened to him," I said.

"Yeah, he's not doing bad for a dog that broke every bone in his body!"

Kismet

SUDDEN WEAKNESS was the only history printed on the form, the only explanation I had for what brought my next case into the Animal Emergency Clinic of the Desert.

It was a Tuesday night, within my first year of employment at the emergency clinic. I was still not terribly confident in my abilities, and I entered the room containing my new Mystery Case with some trepidation.

A twelve-year-old Abyssinian cat lay on the examination table in frustrated parody of a normal Abby's insatiable curiosity. Kismet could not lift her head, and so appeared at first glance to be sniffing the tabletop incessantly. When she tried to take a step forward, she rolled awkwardly on her right shoulder and seemed to have lost track of which way was up.

Sharon followed me into the room. She often did this, in the early days.

My immediate reaction upon seeing the cat's posture was relief. I recognized the syndrome. This would be a quick fix, a chance to look good in the eyes of both the owner and Sharon, the technician I'd been trying to impress for almost a year without notable success.

"She's hypokalemic," I pronounced.

Two blank stares.

"The potassium level in her blood is too low. It weakens the muscles—especially, for reasons that aren't clear, the muscles along the neck and back. It also makes it hard for the nerves to send messages to those muscles, which explains the incoordination."

"But how did she get this way?" her owner asked. She was an assertive middle-aged woman named Sara Albright, and she asked a very good question.

I wished I had a good answer. "We don't know," I had to admit. The ubiquitous "we" meant to imply that no one knew, no one who was publishing, anyway. It wasn't a matter of my personal ignorance. The syndrome had only recently been identified, and I might have missed it altogether if I hadn't been in school at the time. For some reason, usually in cats who were fed a diet designed to acidify the urine, the kidneys' ability to maintain electrolyte balance was impaired. Potassium supplementation resolved the problem. The company manufacturing the food in question has since addressed the problem, and spontaneous hypokalemia is rare now.

Of course, more research has been done since, and some of the mechanisms have been explained. But all I had to work with was the knowledge of the day.

"What do you feed her?" I asked, anticipating the answer. She was well-dressed, appeared affluent. I assumed she would feed her cat a popular premium-brand cat food. Maybe even a prescription diet recommended by her own veterinarian. She surprised me.

"Canned food. Whatever's on sale."

That stopped me, but not for long. Obviously, whatever had most recently been on sale had the same effect on Kismet's kidneys as the prescription food in question. I decided to ignore this piece of the puzzle that seemed not to fit.

I tried to explain what was known to Ms. Albright.

"So what do we do about it?" she asked when I finished.

That part I knew. Or so I thought. "First I'll draw some blood to confirm the low potassium." Today's desktop lab machines that can run a full chemistry panel in ten minutes were not available at the time, but we did have a small analyzer capable—when it was in the mood—of measuring potassium levels. Fortunately, that night it was on its best behavior.

"Then we'll start an IV and put the cat on a mixture of water and electrolytes, with extra potassium added. And of course we'll recheck her blood levels periodically throughout the night." "We" this time meant Sharon and me, who stood by without comment.

For some reason Ms. Albright was reluctant to leave her pet in my care. However, the lab work confirmed my suspicions and it was obvious that Kismet needed something done, so eventually she agreed to the proposed treatment and went home.

Sharon and I got the intravenous catheter in without incident, and started the cat on a potassium-spiked drip. This had to be monitored carefully because, if given too fast or in too large a quantity, potassium—due to its involvement in nerve and muscle function—can stop the heart. However, too low a blood level can have the same effect, which is why the cat needed to be hospitalized in the first place.

And for a while it appeared to do the trick. Kismet's head came up and she uttered a few tentative meows. She weakly explored her cage. Over two hours she gradually improved, until it was time to get her out and recheck her potassium level.

She fought. She didn't want to have blood drawn. Sharon held her down and we got our sample anyway.

And by the time we put her back in her cage, she was in the same condition she'd been in when she first arrived.

"Something's not right," I mumbled, not yet ready to share my misgivings with Sharon.

The lab indicated only a slight improvement.

I pulled up a stool and watched my patient. She was breathing hard after being restrained, which I thought was a fairly extreme reaction. After all, we'd only drawn a tiny sample of blood. It hadn't taken long.

And as I studied her, she rolled onto one side and before my eyes her abdomen expanded. I mean, it was *growing*! "Damn," I said aloud.

Sharon came over to see.

"Let's take an X-ray," I suggested, at a complete loss. There is a condition in dogs wherein the stomach flips over and becomes distended with air. But even that doesn't happen this fast. And, as far as I knew, it never happens in cats.

By the time we finished, but before the film was developed, Kismet's belly was so distended I was afraid it would put pressure on her diaphragm. I grabbed a large syringe and slipped the needle directly through the skin into her stomach. I sucked out almost two hundred cc's—about seven ounces, much greater than the volume I'd given her intravenously—of dark green fluid, which undoubtedly contained all the missing potassium.

But why was it suddenly accumulating in Kismet's stomach?

The X-ray provided part of the answer. A coiled wire seemed to be suspended within the fluid. It looked like the spring from inside a ballpoint pen. But could a cat swallow a pen? And if it was only the spring itself, I thought it would pass on through.

By now it was about one o'clock in the morning.

Ms. Albright was not overjoyed to hear from me.

"Surgery? You want to operate on my cat?"

I explained again what had happened, what I'd seen on the films, what I thought needed to be done. I still had no clue why her stomach had suddenly filled with fluid. "By the way, you're not missing any ballpoint pens, are you? The kind that click."

Total silence on the line. Then, "No, I don't use that kind." Neutral voice. "How much is this going to cost?"

Ah, the question. Once she'd asked, she'd as good as approved it. I gave her an estimate and she agreed. Irritably.

Sharon already had the OR ready. Marty, our graveyard technician at the time, had come in by then, and helped prepare the cat for surgery. I was nervous about the hypokalemia, but didn't see what else I could do.

Oddly, her stomach had not re-expanded. I was past trying to imagine what was happening. I was going in to find out instead.

Kismet's stomach was essentially empty, but for a couple of ounces of the same bile-rich juice. But easily palpable in the pylorus—the area where the stomach joins the first part of the small intestine—I felt a lump. It wasn't a pen, it was only an inch or so long. And it was too substantial to be just the spring.

I cut through the tissue and the object slipped out into my hand. It was nothing I'd ever seen. It was roughly mushroom-shaped, and made of gray-green hard plastic. I handed it to Sharon and asked her to cut it open and make sure there was a spring inside while I sewed up my incision. There was.

"I know what it is!" Marty exclaimed.

We both turned to her.

"It's one of those thermometers they put in turkeys so you know when they're done! See, this top part pops up out of the meat, and when you see it you can take the turkey out and carve it."

After a pause, Sharon agreed that's probably what it was.

I waited until the following morning to tell Ms. Albright what we'd found.

"I'm sure you're mistaken," she said. "I've never had that kind of turkey in my house. In fact, we haven't cooked any sort of turkey for years."

"Well," I said, ready to be convinced, "my tech seems awfully sure. At any rate, Kismet is doing fine and she's ready to be transferred to your regular vet." The emergency clinic was closed between eight and five on weekdays, and we tried not to leave animals unobserved during that time.

Ms. Albright seemed relieved at that. She showed up promptly at seven-thirty, but by the time she arrived she'd figured everything out.

"The cat food I bought last month was all turkey flavored," she said. "I'm sure that's where the thermometer came from."

And she was right. It turns out that much pet food is made from cast-off human food. In this case, turkey. The *whole* turkey! The entire carcasses are boiled down to mush, then pressed into cans.

Ms. Albright was a lawyer. She contacted the cat food company that same day. Her combined vet bills came to around twelve hundred dollars.

The cat food company paid every cent.

Della

The mastiff puppy my mother gave me for graduation learned to adapt. We lived, however briefly, at my mother's goat farm; in a condo, a house, and a duplex in northern California; a trailer behind the equine hospital; then a roomy, nearly unfurnished house while I worked at the equine hospital; on five acres in Morongo Valley for two years; then back to town when I bought a small house with a big yard in Palm Springs. Sometimes we had roommates; my roommates usually had dogs. Della played gently with anyone she could find. She went to work with me almost every day during my internship and later at the emergency clinic. She lived to please me. She was an exceptional companion.

When she was two, I bred her to a champion mastiff from Riverside. She produced six puppies, of which I kept a male. His name is Moby. I spayed her soon after, and neutered Moby. Della finally had a permanent playmate, but taking the two of them to work became a bit impractical. I didn't mind leaving them home. They had each other.

When we moved "down the hill" to Palm Springs, my "new" house required a lot of work. Contractors came and went. I knocked out a wall, ripped up carpets and replaced them, stripped and painted the plaster walls, and completely remodeled the kitchen.

For most of this time the dogs opted to stay outside. It was spring and the weather was fine. The huge yard—my house's best feature—was surrounded by a high wooden fence. It wasn't five acres like I had in Morongo, but there was plenty of room to play. Della adjusted better than Moby did; Moby had only known open space. But they seemed content and I was wrapped up in my project. So when Della first began losing weight I barely noticed.

Then one day she vomited. I took a good look at her, for the first time in months. I was shocked and ashamed to note how thin she was. I took her to the clinic and ran blood work, which revealed liver disease. X-rays, then a barium series—not easy on even a thin mastiff—told me her spleen was enlarged as well.

We'd had a tick problem in Morongo. The desert is proof against most fleas, mosquitoes and other parasites, but ticks flourish. This was before some of the new products that effortlessly kill the repulsive things. Frequent tick baths and dips helped, but I could not exterminate five acres.

Ticks in certain arid zones of the country carry a rickettsial organism called Ehrlichia canis. A distant cousin to Rocky Mountain spotted fever, E. canis was a gift from Vietnam, courtesy of the military canine corps. Transmitted from dog to dog by various tick species, it can cause a disease called Tropical Pancytopenia. More commonly, we refer to it as simply Ehrlichiosis. The most common finding is bleeding—from the nose, into the urine, almost anywhere. Lab work initially reveals a drastic reduction in the number of circulating platelets, the tiny cell particles that aid in clotting. Della's platelet count was very low. Serum titers later confirmed the infection.

Normally the disease responds well to tetracycline or its derivatives. However, in a few cases, it can cause organ failure. The mechanism for this is probably immune-mediated, or caused by the animal's own immune system as it attempts to eliminate the parasite. Splenomegaly—an enlarged spleen—is common and irrelevant; the elevated liver enzymes and her weight loss were ominous.

I started her on tetracycline and later switched her to doxycycline, a more sophisticated drug. Initially she seemed to do well. The vomiting stopped and she gained a little weight. Her liver enzymes dropped and her platelet count normalized.

Then the vomiting began anew. She developed ascites, or fluid in the abdominal cavity. Her distended belly and bony rib cage made her look like a famine refugee. I drained the fluid and called a specialist I'd referred other cases to in the past. I drove her down to Los Angeles for a long-overdue liver ultrasound and biopsy.

The ultrasound showed a shrinking liver—evidence of severe, irreversible damage. Normal liver tissue was being replaced with scar tissue. Attempts to obtain a noninvasive biopsy were unsuccessful. The needle, seen clearly on the sonogram, repeatedly bounced off the surface of the organ. Della, sedated but awake, began to squirm. She'd been on her back a long time. We gave up and I took her home.

On the way she crashed. We spent the night at the clinic, she on an IV, I stretched out beside her in the run. I began to understand—to *feel*, which is not the same as knowing—how all those clients felt who had insisted on staying with their pets as long as I would let them. Perhaps Della had accepted her death long before, I don't know. But I had yet to believe she wouldn't rally.

I had been at AEC a little over two years at that point. I still relied heavily on other vets' input for major decisions. Bob Rooks, the specialist I'd consulted and who had provided the ultrasound, recommended surgical biopsy. I doubted Della would survive surgery, and, more to the point, I was sure her liver was too far gone. A biopsy would take days of processing time, and would almost certainly reveal scarring and end-stage changes. An enlarged liver has a chance to regenerate. A cirrhotic one does not.

I called Sue Klages, who came over on her lunch break. She took one look at Della and knew what had to be done. I held her while Sue delivered the fatal injection into her IV line. Della never felt a thing.

I have watched Ehrlichiosis wreak havoc with biological systems. Dogs who were diagnosed much earlier than Della have deteriorated and died despite every effort to save them. But others have been pulled from the brink.

I will never know whether my own distraction made the difference. I was afraid of surgery at the time; today I wouldn't hesitate to open a belly much earlier, get the biopsy I needed if I couldn't do so any other way. On that last day it was too late, but I will always wonder if my own denial killed her. She got sick during a period in my life when I simply wasn't paying attention. And at a time when I stood at a professional crossroads—just how far do we go to get the answers?

Della's death served as something of a catalyst. My guilt made me reluctant to talk about it, but it cemented the validity of my career path. If I wavered in the past, not fully grasping the importance of the human/companion animal bond, I now understood it to my core.

On-The-Job Training

Robert M. Miller once drew a cartoon of a fancy car parked in front of a veterinary clinic, indicating somehow that it belonged to the veterinarian. The license plate read: PARVO.

Officially discovered in 1969, the virus—apparently mutated from one that previously infected only cats—still runs rampant. Fortunately, a concerted research effort resulted in the development of a vaccine in record time. Parvo, at least the severe form of the disease, can usually be prevented. But a disheartening number of people either don't know when to vaccinate, or put it off, or simply don't care enough to protect their puppies.

Unfortunately, even vaccinated puppies sometimes come down with the disease. This is especially true during the first three to four months of life, before the immune system has matured enough to fully respond to the vaccine and before the series is completed.

Wherever a reservoir—a population of unvaccinated dogs—remains, the virus will be sustained. There are large geographic pockets in the desert where stray animals abound—pets who have been abandoned or are simply allowed to roam free. These animals lead short, miserable lives, and produce sickly puppies that wind up in under-budgeted shelters. Adopted by well-intentioned families, these pups are taken to veterinarians, groomers, public parks, and the homes of other people who own puppies. By the time they show symptoms they may have infected a dozen other dogs.

The virus is transmitted in feces, one dog to another. It has been shown to survive for over two months in the environment, under ideal conditions. These are proven facts. I believe it can travel great distances on the wind—that is my own theory, unproven but logical. I think it is transferred from one place to another on the soles of shoes and carried by flies as they flit from one pile to the next, oblivious to fences and other boundaries. These ideas are borne out by the fact that clinical cases of parvo increase dramatically during spring and fall.

Spring and fall—puppy season. Mild climate, and, in the desert, wind storms. Parvo season. Some weekends the Emergency Clinic's nine-cage Isolation facility filled up with vomiting, dehydrated puppies. Intravenous fluids drip in; the foulest-smelling bloody diarrhea drips out. Innocent brown eyes reflect misery. Way too many die.

Long ago—had it already been eight years?—as an undergrad I worked briefly in a small-animal clinic near Phoenix. We had treated parvo with intravenous fluids and antibiotics—useless against the virus itself but helpful in combating the secondary infections that moved in opportunistically. In 1989, that was still all we had to offer. And the dogs were still dying.

During vet school, I'd spent a "free block" in Lexington, Kentucky, at a high-profile equine hospital. I'd helped treat a lot of sick foals. One of the things we used a lot of was equine plasma. It contained immunoglobulins—a sort of generic antibody that helped the immature immune system combat microbes.

In certain cases, both for human and veterinary use, horses are hyperimmunized—injected over and over with a specific disease-causing agent until they produce huge quantities of antibody against that disease without becoming ill themselves. This "hyperimmune serum" is then harvested and concentrated for use in emergencies. Examples are tetanus antitoxin and antivenin for snakebite. A new product at the time protected horses against endotoxin, a byproduct of bacterial death that could lead to shock and other fatal side effects.

Why couldn't the same principle be applied to parvo in puppies? Parvoviruses as a group attack the host's immune system directly, destroying the animal's ability to fight off the virus. Thus the high mortality rate. This effect can be demonstrated by monitoring an infected puppy's white blood cell count daily—at the time, we assumed a count below 1,000 (normal ranging around 6–16,000) meant the case was hopeless. I had taken this as gospel. Those would be the puppies I would experiment on first.

The first was a tiny cocker spaniel pup named Winchell, only about six weeks old. Normally that breed survives the disease, but this pup just kept deteriorating. I explained my theory to his owner and got permission to transfuse Winchell.

On the theory that if the white blood cells were being wiped out, more white blood cells were needed, I transfused this pup with whole blood. White cell extract is not available, but fresh whole blood contains white blood cells along with plasma and oxygen-carrying red cells. Within a few hours Winchell was up, wagging his tail, whining for attention. I was thrilled, and so was his owner. We waited to see whether the improvement would hold.

The next day the puppy began to show signs of jaundice. Despite fairly aggressive treatment, he deteriorated and we finally put him to sleep. It may have been the first genuine transfusion reaction I'd ever seen, or it may have been a system shutting down after too much sickness. I'll never know, but it was a bitter disappointment.

The next one was a female rottweiler named Sadie. Rotts, for some reason, are exquisitely sensitive to parvo. This one was three months old, the immune system's most vulnerable stage. She developed signs just as her brother was recovering, after a week of touch-and-go hospitalization. Sadie was not so lucky. Despite the usual fluids and antibiotics, she went downhill quickly.

Again I explained my theory. Again the owner agreed to the experiment. He had nothing to lose. Sadie's response to whole blood transfusion was initially less dramatic, but the next day her white cell count was indeed increased. The day after, it went up some more. Sadie stopped vomiting, and her diarrhea decreased as well. But her appetite never returned. I sent her home after a week, hoping that being reunited with her brother in a familiar environment would help. It did not. Sadie wasted away. A month later I euthanized the emaciated puppy, now faded to a grotesque caricature of herself. Her owner and I were both in tears.

My theory clearly needed revising. Perhaps the cellular portion of the blood was a problem. It was not practical to separate white from red cells for transfusion purposes, and red cells carry antigens that occasionally result in negative reactions. What

I'd seen did not resemble what I'd been taught to expect from such a reaction, but because the puppies' immune systems were so badly compromised, perhaps dealing with foreign cells was simply too much for them. The actual answer is much more complicated, but suffice it to say, the cells were not such a great idea.

Unfortunately, at the time I did not have a source for commercially available canine plasma. We obtained our fresh whole blood from local dogs, usually shelter animals that were considered unadoptable because of aggression problems and slated for euthanasia. The head of one such shelter agreed to help me. She designated two dogs for hyperimmunization, and set them up to be vaccinated against parvo every two weeks for eight weeks. Two weeks after the final injection, I drew the blood into special bags I'd obtained from the human blood bank. By prior arrangement I took the bags back to the blood bank where they were centrifuged and the plasma separated from blood. This I transported on ice back to the clinic, where I froze it in anticipation of the next suitable case.

I didn't have long to wait. A young Australian shepherd mix of uncertain history, almost certainly never vaccinated before (her new owner found her as a stray), came in a few days after I'd collected my precious plasma. She was in terrible shape by the time I saw her, her white count already under 2,000. I discussed the situation with her owner, and we decided to try.

It worked. Maybe she would have lived anyway, but I didn't think so.

It worked on the next one, and the next—both rottweilers. Lost causes, one would have thought, and they went home and thrived. But then I was out of plasma. My contact at the blood bank declined to help me further, citing fear of lawsuits or negative publicity if word got out that canine blood had passed through her facility—despite the rigid labeling we had done and the absolute impossibility of cross-contamination between bags. She was probably right, but it frustrated me.

A colleague in Yucca Valley, John Sexton, had been following these efforts. He apprised me of a commercial canine blood bank in central California. He had obtained fresh-frozen plasma by next-day air, transfused a deteriorating rottweiler puppy and seen the near-miraculous recovery that followed. I contacted

Animal Blood Bank and discovered an unlimited source for fresh-frozen canine plasma.

Plasma, I eventually realized, does more than provide antibody. It contains all the proteins and other life-sustaining chemicals that are busily leaking out through the damaged intestinal mucosa. It carries clotting factors where they are needed, and provides osmotic balance to keep infused fluids in the bloodstream instead of oozing into tissues and the intestinal tract by way of diseased vascular beds.

But it isn't cheap. Over the next year, our average cost for treating a parvo case increased from around three hundred dollars to nearly a thousand. But our survival rate neared ninety-five percent, maybe more—instead of the tossup I'd grown to expect. Parvo became a challenge I looked forward to instead of the dismal prospect it had always been before.

I was not the only person to whom this idea occurred. At conferences I began to hear rumors of new products, including a version of anti-endotoxin serum labeled for dogs. But our clinic's success encouraged me to try new treatments sooner. I had come to the desert under the assumption that all my referring veterinarians knew more than I did, since they were all more experienced. But daytime practice isn't like emergency work. They didn't see the same sort of cases.

It was a lesson I learned over and over again.

All This
For A Dog?

It was the beginning of commitment. Of growing into the job, of pushing a little harder, of refusing to accept a certain mortality rate with a shrug of my shoulders. I had stumbled into a profession that provided for wide-ranging philosophies, and I'd been exposed to many of those. It was time to create my own.

Della's death galvanized me. I could help prevent other animals from dying prematurely, spare other pet owners from watching them die. Every death happened for a reason, and understanding those reasons could bring us closer to life.

High-quality life. I am grateful that we as veterinarians still have the escape hatch of euthanasia, for those cases in which we cannot offer relief from pain or a semblance of normality. Cases that come to mind are spinal fractures with complete loss of function, profound head traumas, refractory kidney failure (though even kidney transplants are now possible). But all too often death is the easy way out, the inexpensive way.

"We can probably save him," I say sometimes, "but it will cost a lot of money. And a lot of time. Your time, once he goes home." "Put him to sleep." It is said through tears, guilt and anger and self-loathing, but the forms are signed and the deed is done. And the people go about their lives and adopt new pets. All those medical skills we learned amount to nothing if owners aren't committed to their pets.

I have no doubt these pet owners experience grief and remorse. But for most of them it's a single event in their lifetime, or one that occurs only rarely. Imagine the veterinarian who knows she has the skill to return these animals to health, but day after day is required to ignore those abilities and kill the patients she was taught to save. Is it any wonder that so many veterinarians leave the profession, burn out or go to human medical school?

Fortunately, I had stumbled into a geographic area where a high proportion of clients are very committed to their pets. This allowed me to push myself, to learn and to practice what I learned.

The parvo experiment empowered me. It was the first time I'd rationalized a treatment protocol that had not been taught to me by someone else. Watching a wriggling, ecstatic puppy leave in its owner's arms, a pup that by all expectation should have been dead, made the long nights worthwhile.

What other conditions might deserve better therapies? Heatstroke? There was almost nothing in the literature about this condition, and what I'd found advised wetting the animal and treating for shock—exactly as we were doing. But virtually all of them developed DIC, a clotting disorder, and subsequently died.

DIC was another condition that had been discussed more thoroughly with regard to horses than dogs, but I knew it affected all mammalian species, including humans. We'd been taught possible treatment regimens, but never given much hope. DIC is the medical abbreviation for Disseminated Intravascular Coagulopathy. But late at night it might as well have meant Dead In Cage, because by the time the animal started bleeding, treatment was a catch-up game that we had little hope of ever winning.

But heatstroke was one situation where we *knew* it would happen. I didn't need to wait for the blood to begin pouring. So, I thought, why not treat preemptively? There were minidoses listed for heparin, doses I recalled giving to horses after colic surgery, doses I found in textbooks for dogs as well. The next case would be given heparin immediately.

As I said, these were dogs who would otherwise die. Unproven treatment could not make things worse.

First, I stuck a few bags of electrolyte solution in the refrigerator. Wetting down a big, overheated dog seemed counterproductive. Once the dog's temperature dropped it tended to keep on dropping, the result being a big, wet, *cold* dog who had no control over its own body temperature. It made more sense to cool them from within.

What else? Good old plasma—which I found myself using more and more, for liver disease, shock, pancreatitis, any condition in which the body's own protein equilibrium was severely disrupted. Certainly it was the only definitive treatment for active DIC. All that damaged tissue could only benefit from transfusion. Not to mention those lost clotting factors.

I planned it out. I was ready. I waited.

Fortunately, most desert dwellers know better than to leave pets unattended in cars, or staked outside without water and shade, or to allow them to exercise too strenuously on a hot day. But we still see the occasional dog who was jogging with its owner and hit a point of no return, where they simply cannot cool themselves in the usual way. Most cases, however, belong to visitors.

The first one was a boxer named Frannie. A disproportionate number of heatstroke cases are boxers. This one had been left with the owner's daughter while she traveled. The owner lived in central California, where it was probably twenty degrees cooler. But the daughter, whose name was Ann, had a wading pool and doggy door for her own dog. She made sure Frannie knew where both were that first morning, and headed off to work.

Who knows what went through Frannie's mind? When she brought the dog in to AEC that evening, Ann said, "I got home from work about five-twenty. The dogs were outside, but when I got to the kitchen Frannie came in through the doggy door and collapsed. She could have come inside any time! How did this happen?"

I had no answer for that. But I did have treatment for Frannie. Her temperature when she arrived was 112 degrees. We treated her exactly as I'd planned. And she did great. No bloody diarrhea, no rebound hypothermia. Just a steady recovery.

Of course I was not the only one who ever thought of these things. But little hard research had been done so the results were not published. I could not open a text and find this treatment protocol outlined in writing. I felt alone, casting about in the dark, discovering gems but having no idea what I might be missing.

Knowledge of emergency and critical care both in human and veterinary medicine was exploding. New drugs and new combinations of old drugs made it possible to save animals that would previously have died. New technologies put diagnostic tools in our reach that had formerly been prohibitively expensive. Every few months something new and previously unimaginable became real and doable.

Before I was officially Director of AEC, the board allowed us to purchase state-of-the-art laboratory and X-ray equipment. This improved our services dramatically. Both paid for themselves the first year they were in place. We upgraded from halothane to isoflurane anesthesia, newly approved for animals and safer for the compromised animals we were called upon to anesthetize. We added IV pumps and oxygen concentrators—reconditioned castoffs from human hospital suppliers. We bought a pulse oximeter to monitor anesthesia quickly and easily. A client who worked at a local hospital brought us cast-off equipment for a fraction of their usual cost: ECG telemetry, syringe pumps, a better lab centrifuge, eventually an endoscope and a temperature monitor. I became expert at tracking down used equipment and bargaining for their purchase. Electrolyte and blood gas measuring capabilities greatly expanded our lab services. A computerized ECG analyzing system eliminated the delay in cardiac evaluation.

Within a couple of years, our spacious clinic was crowded. Every spare inch of wall space was lined with equipment. And all of it was used regularly.

I joined the Veterinary Emergency and Critical Care Society. Their biennial convention, held in concert with the College of Veterinary Emergency and Critical Care, which certified specialists in the field, was held on even-numbered years in San Antonio. In 1992 I attended my first. I returned home energized.

I'd been laboring more or less alone in my isolated little corner of the desert, struggling to deal better with certain specific medical conditions as they occurred. The veterinarians who referred their clients rarely saw the emergencies—and when they came, they were intrusions on the ordered schedule of their busy days. They were appreciative but not really interested.

Here, then, was an entire convention hall full of like-minded DVMs. Pale, owl-eyed night people whose main passion in life seemed to be pulling sick animals back from the brink of death. A world opened up before me. If my colleagues at home considered my measures extreme at times, what would they make of discussions of long-term mechanical ventilation, of serial blood gas monitoring, of maintaining surgically implanted feeding tubes for six months or more?

Many—if not most—of the human beings in this world do not have access to the kind of medical care we were discussing. I recall a physician who came to the clinic one Sunday with his father. This was soon after we had sent peacekeeping forces to Somalia. This man had been part of the Red Cross medical team. He wandered our veterinary clinic, taking in the machines, the clean linens, the medical records. "There is more medical equipment in this animal clinic," he told me, "than in the entire country of Somalia." I wasn't sure how to respond to that—a bit of pride mingled with despair, and a certain degree of defensiveness.

Even colleagues have criticized me for going too far. "Those young vets get a little carried away," one referring DVM told a client. I'd been up all night with the client's dog. It had come in on a stretcher and walked out to the car the next morning. It was improving and might have gone home in a few days from the DVM's office, where I was required to send it for more treatment—or it may have deteriorated and died despite our efforts. We'll never know, because the DVM put it to sleep within minutes of its arrival.

Other people have been more blunt. "All this for a dog?" is not an uncommon question. The answer is, "Why not?" Our— the veterinary community's—ability to provide excellent care does not prevent any client from declining that care. No government subsidies or pet Medicare exists. We are capitalism in its purest form—we can provide our service only so long as people are willing to pay us what it costs to provide it. These services grow increasingly expensive as they grow more sophisticated.

Despite all we can offer, some people still ask me to kill their pets for nothing more than a broken leg. The option is always there, hovering like a dark cloud between my patient and me. The good stuff is for the animals lucky enough to be priorities in their owners' lives (and budgets).

And for me.

Who Was Right?

Rorick the cat was brought in for euthanasia. Yet there was enough doubt in John Frank's mind that he wanted his old Siamese cat looked at first. I entered the room with no idea what was coming.

Rorick was eighteen years old. His blue irises were faded and atrophied into a lacy network that only hinted at their former glory. He weighed about four pounds; Mr. Frank assured me he had never been over ten. When I picked up a fold of skin it stayed folded—a sign of severe and chronic dehydration. Yet he squinted his eyes and leaned into my fingers when they brushed his cheek.

Mr. Frank was about forty. Rorick had come to him as a kitten. That meant he had owned this cat for almost half his life. The tears that threatened to escape down his cheeks were quite understandable. At any rate, they were nothing new to me. But he was not ready for me to take the cat and disappear into the back room. Nor did he want to hold him while I administered the injection. It was a quiet night and I didn't mind chatting with him about his once-regal cat.

"He was a wedding gift from my wife," he said.

I hesitated to ask if they were still married. They were.

"Has he been sick long?" I asked, unconsciously noting the expensive clothes and casual authority with which Mr. Frank carried himself.

"I took him in to my vet because of this pus in his eyes," he said. His voice became clearer. Talking helped. But I didn't see any pus—only the mucus that accumulates when the body is too dried out to produce tears.

"What did your vet say?"

"That he has kidney failure and there's nothing we can do. "He said he was going to die soon."

I bit my tongue. I assumed treatment options had been discussed and declined.

"Then he gave him a cortisone shot for the eye infection."

A red flag raised itself in my mind. Corticosteroids aren't the treatment of choice for any infection—in many cases, they are strongly contraindicated. This is basic medical knowledge.

Steroids are also a bad idea in the face of renal failure—they tend to blunt the already suppressed ability of the kidneys to retain water. In other words, a "cortisone" shot would tend to worsen existing dehydration. Besides, I saw no indication of any eye infection to begin with. Either this client had gotten it very wrong, or his vet had let him down spectacularly.

"What was her BUN?" I asked, referring to a basic blood test for renal function. Blood Urea Nitrogen, or BUN, is a toxin that healthy kidneys eliminate from the body. Even in hospitals that lack lab equipment, a crude version of this test can be done on an inexpensive paper strip that changes color based on BUN concentration.

"Her what?"

"Didn't your vet do some blood work before he diagnosed the kidney failure?" By now my incredulity must have been obvious, despite my effort at keeping my voice neutral. I always tried to reserve judgment when I disagreed with what clients told me their veterinarians had said or done. So often there are two very different sides to the story. But this man didn't even know you could do blood work on cats.

"What treatment options did he discuss with you?"

"He just told me there wasn't any treatment. Rorick hasn't been eating, and he's lost so much weight. He just said I'd know when it was time to put him to sleep."

This put me in a tough spot. Without local veterinarians referring cases, the emergency clinic would not exist. However, this client had, in my opinion, been severely cheated by his vet. It certainly would not have been wrong to euthanize this cat—it was so clearly dying. But I'd seen animals in much worse shape, from renal failure or other diseases, respond to treatment and live months or even years of good quality life.

I was still petting Rorick. "Well, he may be right, but I personally have a different philosophical perspective," I said carefully. "Of course, if you want to put him down that wouldn't be wrong—he looks pretty bad. But he's terribly dehydrated and worn out from not eating, and those are things we can correct. His body temperature is below normal, and sometimes just warming them up makes them feel better. And blood work may reveal an electrolyte abnormality, which can result in weakness. At this point we don't even know for sure it *is* kidney failure."

Despite my caution, Mr. Frank was picking up on my dismay. I'd told him the exact truth, as I saw it. Chances were, the renal failure diagnosis was correct—it's the most common illness in geriatric cats. If so, no matter what was done, Rorick's disease would eventually kill him. The other vet had decided, in his own mind, that Rorick wasn't worth treating. And many clients would agree with that.

But I was looking at a man who loved his cat. He was an intelligent, educated person who could afford treatment had it been suggested. He should have been included in the decision whether to treat his cat or not.

Treatment is available—not a cure, but many levels of treatment ranging from supportive rehydration to dialysis. For cats who qualify, kidney transplants are available! The more practical therapies are time-consuming and sometimes frustrating, because not every animal responds favorably. But failing to even offer to treat—or worse, giving treatment that might actually worsen the problem—was, in my mind, unconscionable. No veterinarian has any business making unilateral decisions in these cases. I don't know whether this involved laziness, miscommunication, arrogance, rank incompetence, burnout, or some combination thereof. But the vet in question had failed his client in a big way.

I had only to mention other possibilities, and Mr. Frank was all for treatment. Within a short time, Rorick had lab work, an IV line, and a nasogastric tube to deliver liquid nutrients to his shriveled stomach. He languished in our incubator for nearly a week—Mr. Frank and I were in agreement that he should not return to the other hospital, and I had informed the board of directors what was happening. Rorick did, in fact, suffer from renal failure, and virtually every possible complication that involved. He was anemic, with severe electrolyte abnormalities that failed to stabilize for days.

Over time, his body temperature increased and his hydration status improved markedly. He gained almost a pound. He received antibiotics, potassium, anti-ulcer drugs, and a synthetic hormone to stimulate his bone marrow and correct the anemia. He received appetite stimulants and daily visits from his owner.

The rapport between Rorick and his owner was amazing to behold. Once he felt better, the cat would march gracefully up Mr. Frank's arm, chattering and complaining constantly the way Siamese cats do. He would perch on his owner's shoulder and speak into his ear.

The change in Mr. Frank was fascinating as well. The night I met him, he was guarded and grieving. He now clearly looked forward to his visits, and some of the guilt was gone. I say guilt because that's what pet owners feel when they make hasty decisions involving euthanasia. It's there anyway, to some extent, but it helps to know you've tried everything reasonably possible. And no one could doubt that Rorick was getting better.

But he wouldn't eat. We could feed him all we wanted, dripping the milklike diet through the tube that snaked down one nostril and into his stomach. He wasn't even aware of its presence. And occasionally, when a bit of baby food was placed in his mouth, he would swallow it. Otherwise all offerings went ignored. Something inside Rorick had decided it was time to die, and he wasn't putting out any effort to change that course.

We tried gourmet cat foods, chicken and fish and shrimp and baby food. We gave drugs known to stimulate the appetite. We tried removing the feeding tube, thinking its presence might interfere with swallowing. Mr. Frank came in and sat with his cat and tempted him with all sorts of goodies. Nothing worked.

He did, however, begin to take water. We decided to send him home to see if the familiar environment helped.

For another week he hung out in front of the refrigerator, where the warm air blew out from underneath. He drank a little water and he continued to refuse his favorite foods. His body temperature dropped again.

Then the Franks had to leave town for three days, on a trip

that had been planned for months. Rorick came back. This time, Mr. Frank realistically declined the life-sustaining measures we had used before. Rorick lived in the incubator but received his fluids under the skin. We force-fed him three times daily but did not replace the feeding tube. He grew more depressed without Mr. Frank's visits.

When Mr. Frank returned, he saw his pet with fresh eyes. The once-vibrant Siamese crouched apathetically in a corner of his enclosure. He no longer climbed his owner's arm or sat on his shoulder—he was too weak even if he wanted to try. With tears in his eyes, Mr. Frank once again signed the form requesting euthanasia for Rorick. This time he stayed. His companion of eighteen years died in his arms.

Years later, I think about Rorick when I am tempted to push a client toward treatment or away from it. Who was right? The vet who "knew" it was no use, or the one who tried and failed? There is no answer. Mr. Frank clearly felt better for having tried; the cost of treatment was never an issue. However, when he began to realize our efforts were for naught, he may have believed that postponing euthanasia only prolonged his pet's misery.

I have treated other cats—and dogs—with the same condition, in even worse shape, with excellent results. Others, like this one, simply do not respond. So much depends on the patient, and intangible factors such as the animal's will to live.

It's possible that, had treatment been initiated sooner, Rorick might have responded. It's equally possible he had simply given up and accepted his own inevitable death, and nothing anyone could do would have made the slightest difference.

No one can know what any given animal is feeling. As pet owners, we are charged with making decisions for them based on our own, often strongly anthropomorphized, sense of how we would feel in their place. These decisions are also influenced by financial considerations, guilt, family pressure ("My husband never did like Blackie. I've had this dog longer than we've been married."), and personal loss.

Every veterinarian has his or her own value system, which enters the equation. We are human; we can't help it. By definition we are people who chose to enter a profession whose rewards are more often emotionally than financially gratifying.

Some seem motivated more by money or the personal sense of accomplishment associated with pulling off a difficult save. Others appear baffled and intimidated by the technological advancements that have occurred since they graduated; it is almost impossible to keep up with all of these, so they are rejected as extreme or unnecessary. Clients are denied referral to specialists because they never learn it exists.

And, to paraphrase, we bury the evidence of our ignorance.

Stormy's
Miracle

The first time I met Stuart Gilmore I didn't think his cat had a chance.

Stormy lay unconscious on the exam table, a rack of bones with a loose filthy hide draped over it. Her sunken eyes and prominent cheekbones told me she was ancient. She did not respond in any way to my probings and manipulations.

"How old is she?" I asked with the automatic professional sympathy that crept into my voice when I knew I'd be euthanizing an animal I just met.

"I'm not sure. I found her about twelve years ago, and she wasn't a kitten then."

I was surprised. Despite her emaciation, I had taken Stormy for a purebred Burmese. She had the large ears and fine bone structure; a long slender tail tucked stiffly against her body as if for warmth; short, once-sleek brown fur now matted and unkempt. "How long has she been sick?"

He considered. "As far as I know, she was okay yesterday. But I didn't realize she'd gotten this thin. Sometimes it's hard to keep track."

"Has she been eating?"

A helpless shrug. "I have a lot of cats."

I understood. The food disappears. Who can say which cats ate and which didn't? "How many?" Idle conversation.

He had to think about it. "Seventeen," he finally said, but without assurance. Then, more confidently: "Seventeen."

That was, I agreed, a lot of cats. I'd had clients with more—Mrs. Willery came to mind, a woman who collected cats like trading stamps, and had passed the fifty mark last time I spoke to her. She called often, hoping for free advice. She believed amoxicillin cured everything. But her cats were half-wild, unneutered and were taken in with misguided compassion, the result being frequent outbreaks of viral infections in the unvaccinated horde. Then there was Mrs. Oldenham, with fifty or sixty dogs, and a paid staff to take care of them. Those dogs got the best of care, and I knew she'd set up a trust fund to keep them going after her death.

I didn't know which end of the spectrum Mr. Gilmore belonged on. He was quiet and unassuming. He wore a faded polo shirt and khakis that hung on his hips like an afterthought. His white hair was of no particular length or style. He drove up in an old station wagon. He lived right there in Thousand Palms. The carrier in which Stormy had arrived was filthy. And yet, he spoke like an educated man. He had recently retired, bought a patch of land and was building a house on it. In the meantime, he lived on it in a mobile home with his cats.

"Please do whatever you can for her," he said.

"It gets very expensive," I warned. "And her odds aren't good. Once they're this sick, it's a race against time to get the right diagnosis, and it may still be too late." It had been two years since Rorick Frank, but this case reminded me of that one. Professional challenge warred against the frustration of pulling out all stops and failing anyway.

"If she has any chance at all, I'd like to see that she gets it." He was firm without being pushy. Accepting but not fatalistic.

So we would treat. It was early Sunday morning; that gave me twenty-four hours to do what I could. Jane wrote up an estimate while I ran lab work and Rebecca got Stormy situated in the incubator with an IV line. Mr. Gilmore left a credit card deposit. Before he left I reiterated the poor prognosis. Mr. Gilmore again insisted that he wanted everything done for his Stormy.

It was one of the most involved cases I've ever handled. Stormy was negative on all the virus assays, which came as a relief. Her kidneys were failing, yes—but the numbers weren't high enough to explain the coma. Ditto her electrolytes—not normal by any means, but not that bad either.

She was critically anemic, meaning an absence of the red blood cells that carry oxygen to the tissues. "Tired blood," it's often called, because of the symptoms of anemia in humans. The normally red blood is watery and resembles weak cherry Kool-Aid. A blood smear revealed high numbers of immature red cells, indicating regeneration, or an attempt by the bone marrow to replace the missing cells. The failing kidneys were not at fault in this case.

Stripped to basics, the causes of anemia are three: loss, as in bleeding, whether slow or fast; destruction, as in autoimmune disease; or bone marrow suppression, in which case the cells are not being manufactured fast enough to make up for those lost to normal turnover. So far we'd ruled out only this last one. The young cells indicated a supercharged bone marrow. So we anesthetized Red, the clinic blood donor, and drew blood for a transfusion.

Mr. Gilmore reported having lost another cat to cancer within the past year, but thought that cat had also been anemic. He couldn't recall the name of the disease, but it was an infection that caused anemia, he said.

I thought about a parasite called Hemobartonella. I hadn't seen a case since vet school—it was rare in the desert. But this cat had recently moved from Los Angeles. I didn't see any indication of parasitism on a blood smear, but started her on doxycycline anyway.

She was crawling with fleas; fleas live by drinking the blood of their hosts. Were there enough to explain the severity of her anemia? I didn't know; at any rate they weren't helping. We bathed her and combed out the mostly dead parasites. Stormy was, by then, already regaining consciousness.

A nasogastric tube provided nourishment; the IV added blood, then electrolytes and fluid. She got oxygen and warmth from the incubator. Mr. Gilmore seemed satisfied by the number of tubes converging on his pet. He might not understand the specific purpose of each, but they were evidence that we had taken him at his word. We were clearly doing everything we could to help Stormy.

Mr. Gilmore didn't have a regular veterinarian yet; he asked me for a recommendation. I knew that few local clinics were prepared to deal with so sick a patient. At the time I was considering a partnership with Nancy Carlson in the Palm Desert clinic she managed and eventually bought. I suggested he take Stormy there.

More tests. She was up now, walking around the cage, beginning to take baby food. The anemia had been corrected with the transfusion; we never did learn its cause. She gained weight—partly due to rehydration, but calories helped, too.

Stormy went home later that week. The cat I was convinced should be put to sleep went home purring and grooming herself. By then she was like any geriatric cat with renal failure, and renal failure was something we could manage. Mr. Gilmore's bill was over two thousand dollars, but he never complained. We never found out why Stormy was so sick that morning, but she'd gotten better anyway.

Stormy lived another eight months. Eventually she died of complications associated with hypertension, or high blood pressure. It's a common sequela to renal failure. Nancy kept me posted on the case.

Stormy's case reinforced two important ideas. One: Don't prejudge clients. Give every client every option, and let him or her make the decision. And two: Every patient, as long as it is not in intractable pain, deserves a chance.

An Eye For Trouble
(Or, When In Doubt,
Ask Someone Who Knows!)

So many of the worst cases happen on a holiday.

In Dolly's case it was New Year's Eve. It was her eye. And her owners were frantic.

A scratch or puncture had been seen previously. Her regular veterinarian had, a few days earlier, prescribed a standard antibiotic ointment, but the infection had not responded. The ulcer grew in width and depth until the cornea—the clear part of the eye that separates its liquid contents from the outside world—was nearly ruptured. A disconcerting bulge was visible where the thin basement membrane threatened to give way.

Dolly was a sweet-natured Lhasa apso, tolerating my examination with little complaint despite the obvious pain the eye caused her. Her owners, two middle-aged men named Hal and Burt, had not realized how severe the problem was. They only knew it had gotten worse instead of better since treatment began, and it needed to be looked at again.

They were not expecting what I had to say.

"This is what's called a desmetocoele. The surface of the eye has been eaten away, down to a thin layer called Desmete's membrane. That's what's bulging out through the hole." I showed them what I meant. Sure enough, protruding from the uniform roundness of the anterior surface of Dolly's eye was an alarming whitish bubble.

"I don't know whether she's simply got an infection that's resistant to the antibiotics in the medicine she's on. But we don't have time to experiment. I want you to take her to a specialist immediately. A veterinary ophthalmologist."

They exchanged glances and nodded. "Where do we find one?" Hal asked.

"Los Angeles or San Diego."

"We live in LA. We're up here for the holiday. But for Dolly we can certainly go home early."

"Okay, let me make a few calls and find out who's around."

Easier said than done. I suppose one of the attractive things about eye specialization is the dearth of true emergencies. Increasingly desperate, I went down the list, gradually expanding the geographic range. I got answering machines, I got services. Not one doctor was even on call. Many were out of town. New Year's was on a Friday; no one was available until the following Monday. I tried the large referral hospitals, hoping at least for a surgeon; even they had only skeletal staffs.

I knew the ideal treatment for Dolly's eye would involve surgical grafting of a flap of tissue over the defect in her cornea. It was a delicate, tedious operation best done under an operating microscope—but possible with the binocular loupe we had. Should it be done on an infected eye? I wasn't sure. The tissue surrounding the defect looked so friable I didn't want to touch it. I doubted it would hold a suture, even if I was crazy enough to try.

I went back to the exam room, where my clients waited patiently. "There's not a veterinary ophthalmologist even on call in the whole state, as far as I can tell," I said. "If I could just get one on the phone I could at least get advice for temporary management." I looked at the eye again. It looked as if it would burst if she blinked hard. If no one was available, I would have to do my best. But we had only a limited choice of eye medications on hand, and I suspected none would have a broad enough spectrum for this.

Corneal ulcers are common. I see them all the time, and most respond readily to fairly minimal treatment. At the other extreme, a ruptured cornea is a no-brainer: The eye has to be removed, unless it's a small enough, clean enough, fresh enough puncture to sew back up. Even desmetocoeles weren't that unusual, but this was by far the largest one I'd ever seen. That thin membrane isn't meant to hold in the pressure of all that fluid, and the infection that eroded the more superficial layers of tissue was already at work on this last barrier. Whoever treated it got one chance. I did not want to be the one to screw it up.

I really needed a specialist. And it occurred to me that, if I couldn't find a DVM, I would have to try an MD.

A few phone calls told me there was one human ophthalmologist on call for the entire Coachella Valley. His answering service promised to page him, but couldn't say when he would return my call.

I explained the situation to Hal and Burt, and they settled down to wait for the call. Another case came in, I treated it and sent it home. Finally the phone rang. I cannot recall the name of that MD who called me from a restaurant on his cell phone, but his generous advice undoubtedly saved Dolly's eye.

"No, if it's infected it won't hold sutures, and a flap would only seal the infection in. You'll need to debride the margins of the ulcer very carefully with a small blade, then reinforce the cornea. It sounds like she needs Cipro drops and a patch."

"Third eyelid flap?" I asked. Eye patches aren't real practical in dogs.

"As long as it's something you can open and reexamine the eye on a daily basis."

"Cipro . . . I know that's a broad-spectrum antibiotic." It was relatively new, and not approved for veterinary use, but we had its cousin, Baytril. I was wondering if I needed to find a formula for mixing the drops myself. "Does that come in an ophthalmic solution?"

"Yes, of course." There was a pause while we both thought about the differences in our professions. "I don't know where you'll find a pharmacy open today," he finally added. "What do you have on hand?"

We decided on oral Baytril and another topical until a pharmacy opened the next day. I checked with the local hospital just in case, but again met with a machine at the pharmacy. I was sure someone was there for emergencies, but no one was answering the phone.

Once more I updated my clients, and explained our new plan. They were understandably anxious, but appreciative of my efforts. They left Dolly with me.

Under anesthesia, I carefully scraped away at the edges of the defect with a number 15 blade, the smallest scalpel blade on hand. The tissue is surprisingly tough and gives under pressure, so it's actually difficult to perforate a healthy cornea. Even this very diseased one resisted my efforts. But it was important to eliminate as much dead matter as possible, both to remove a barrier to healing and to stimulate the surrounding tissues, in effect reminding the body it had a wound to close.

I knew I'd learned all this at one time. Maybe I should have automatically known how to handle the situation, but I was grateful for the advice I'd received. And Cipro drops sounded like a good thing to know about in any case.

I instilled chloramphenicol ointment over the corneal surface—the best I could do for now—and performed what's called a third eyelid flap. This fairly common technique pulls the tight membrane up from the inside of the eye and holds it against the corneal surface. The suture is pulled through the upper lid and tied in a bow, with a button or piece of tubing to keep it from cutting through the skin. Thus the bulging membrane is gently pushed back in place, dramatically reducing the strain on the paper-thin layer.

Hal and Burt brought Dolly back both Saturday and Sunday, and each day the eye looked a little better. Monday they returned to Los Angeles and their regular vet referred them to an ophthalmologist, who was presumably well-rested from her long weekend off. The ophthalmologist was impressed with what we'd done, they said. "She said, 'I would have managed this eye the exact same way!' "

Dolly is my patient now—her owners eventually made the desert their permanent home. Dolly's cornea has a large permanent scar and still requires periodic visits to the specialist. But Dolly unquestionably sees out of both eyes.

And as she left, I'd swear she winked at me.

Remington Wool

Among the many veterinarians in the desert was a 1987 Kansas graduate named Virginia Skinner. She had gone to work at The Living Desert, our then-small local zoo, upon finishing vet school. I can't remember why she originally called me, but it soon became clear we had a lot in common, having grown up in the Midwest.

I began volunteering at The Living Desert, an experience I never expected to have. Volunteer work is both commitment-free and strangely obligating. I amputated broken raptor wings, removed a tumor from a diamondback's back, palpated a Grevy's zebra for pregnancy (not so easy lying on your side behind an anesthetized beast!), cuddled a tame badger, transfused a baby gazelle. I had the advantage of the emergency work and my previous jobs under supervision. Virginia had connections within the zoo world—so different from practice—but moving directly from school to being the only veterinarian on staff deprived her of experience. We made a good team.

Nevertheless, it didn't last. Virginia moved on to better-paying practice positions, and I found my time more and more limited. Her father died and she moved back to Kansas. Nancy Carlson signed on with The Living Desert on a part-time contract. She was an excellent choice, highly conscientious and experienced in both large- and small-animal practice.

One Saturday afternoon she brought me a lamb. This was not just any adorable baby ruminant, but a bighorn ram lamb. "This is Remington. He's been going downhill for three days. He's not eating. I got the catheter in yesterday, and he feels better with fluids. But I think he's got a hairball."

Hairball. As in what cats vomit onto the white carpet. I studied the broad forehead, the lip curled into perpetual mischievousness, the bright, intelligent eyes dulled by illness. He weighed less than twenty pounds; the nubs above his ears bore little resemblance to the majestic horns they promised.

"What makes you think so?" I asked, skeptical as always.

"He's been totally bottle-fed his entire life" (which amounted to about a month). "He does what foals and calves do, he flank-sucks. I think in the wild, their mothers probably groom them. But since he doesn't have a mom either to remove his loose hair or for him to nurse on, he sucks on his own flanks instead." She pointed to his right flank, where the wool was shorter and sparser than over the rest of his body.

Well, it did make sense. Baby ungulates—animals with hooves—normally stand and nurse shortly after birth. They see well, and many of their cues are visual. Instinctively they look for their mothers' flank, knowing they will find nourishment there. I'd watched enough foals nuzzle and nibble until, half by accident, they latched onto a teat and found sustenance. I'd also seen them get confused at the sight of their own flanks, and briefly suckle themselves. This is unrewarding behavior and normally ceases once they've figured out how to do it right.

"Anyway," Nancy said, "I've given him oil twice, and fluids through the IV and by stomach tube, but it isn't helping. I want you to help me get some X-rays."

That was proper treatment for an intestinal impaction. But a hairball jammed in just the right place could easily prove resistant to lubricants.

Weakened by three days without food, Remington did not struggle much as Nancy removed him from his crate and lifted him onto the X-ray table. We managed to take standing lateral films, so as not to have to hold him in an unnatural position on his side or back. The films confirmed a round mass, containing sand that showed up well, somewhere in one of his four stomach chambers.

That's right, four. Ruminants aren't like other animals. These are the cud-chewers, who chew their partially digested food repeatedly, and with the aid of special bacteria in their rumens—the first, huge chamber—are able to digest tough, fibrous plants that are useless even to most herbivores. Though exquisitely adapted to life on the boulder-strewn mountains that bordered our valley, even a bighorn could not digest his own hair. And all those stomach chambers made surgery difficult; positioning him on his back would predispose him both to organ displacement and regurgitation—something ruminants did naturally but a potential disaster under anesthesia. And this hairball would have to be surgically removed.

Nancy laughed. "That's why I brought him here. You've got the staff, and I want to know everything possible was done to save him."

She wasn't just covering her butt—Nancy wasn't like that. I'd have wanted help, too, in her position. Sheep as a group don't handle surgery well, and this was an inbred, exotic species. Neither of us had operated on a ruminant's abdomen since vet school. Maybe that was just as well—more experienced people might have decided he didn't have a chance.

"Let's do it," I said.

He was small enough to restrain for a mask, so we used only isoflurane to put him under. The techs positioned him on the table and prepped his belly while Nancy and I scrubbed in at the crowded sink. With two of us, things went quickly. The anatomy was unfamiliar, though the huge rumen was unmistakable. We started there, following the path food would take. "Rumen, then reticulum, right?"

"Right. It's the one from anatomy class with the honeycomb, remember?"

She laughed again. "No. That was years ago! This is like The Three Stooges Do Vet Surgery!"

I had to laugh, too. I didn't even own a book detailing this kid's anatomy. "Well, I know that's the order they go in because the last two were omasum and aboma—— what's this?"

"This" was a firm clump of material the size of a large marble, wedged in the narrow opening between the omasum and abomasum—the third and fourth stomach chambers. The abomasum is known as the "true stomach," and felt more familiar.

"Can I just make an incision over the obstruction?" I asked Nancy.

"Don't ask me! You're the surgeon."

I shrugged, and cut just below the mass. I didn't know what

sort of sphincter I might be interrupting if I cut right over it. This made it slightly more difficult, since I had to reach in with hemostats and pull the material out. I handed it to Nancy and began to close the tiny incision in the abomasum.

"Tah-dum!" she said, pulling the mess apart in the sink. "Hair. And sand. Oh, and oil too!" (meaning the mineral oil she'd given him to try to lube the thing through).

"Did you notice how still everything was when we got in?"

"Well, no. But now that you mention it. . . ."

"Look!" I finished stitching the stomach. "His whole gut is moving already!"

"Wow!" It was true—the mass of stomachs and intestines had been gray and virtually still. Now it was a healthy-looking pink, and roiling like a nest of snakes.

"Think we cured him?"

"He's still got to wake up and eat," I pointed out. I started sewing his belly back together.

With a touch of Banamine for pain and endotoxemia, little Remington recovered smoothly. He could be expected to remain depressed for another twenty-four hours, but we watched him closely for signs of pneumonia or other deterioration that might indicate aspiration. None appeared.

After a few hours, Remmy went home with his keeper. He'd been living in her house until he was big enough to wean, so I knew he'd be watched closely. But I was sorry I wouldn't be the one to do it.

The next day Nancy called. "He's chewing his cud!"

"That's great!" I said. It meant his rumen was working again, which was crucial to his recovery.

That night: "He took his bottle!"

The next morning: "He's nibbling hay!"

The following evening: "Susie wants us to put him back the way he was before surgery! This afternoon he jumped over the child barrier she put at the bottom of the stairs to keep him in the living room. He ran up the stairs into the bathroom. Then he grabbed the end of the toilet paper roll and went tearing back downstairs again, and there's toilet paper everywhere!"

I laughed with her. The image was irresistible. "At least toilet paper is soluble! If he eats it, it will just dissolve!"

"Yeah, I guess it beats eating wool. Anyway, Susie's going to be grooming him to minimize the amount of loose wool."

Remington was clearly on his way to a full recovery.

Today he can be seen ruling his harem from the very peak of Bighorn Mountain, the sheep exhibit at The Living Desert. He's a tall, regal ram with the classic scrolled horns that mark the species. But I still remember him as an adorable, mischievous lamb with a penchant for toilet paper and his own wool.

A Little Golden Dog

His owner had to carry him in. He was a golden mutt, maybe cocker spaniel and golden retriever, maybe sheltie and Lab. Maybe a little of everything, with something smaller thrown in for size. He looked to be around eight months old. His eyes held the deep concern of an animal who cannot breathe well, and his hind legs lay limply on the exam table.

It was about six A.M. I'd been up late performing a Caesarean on a cocker spaniel, and I hadn't had my first cup of coffee yet. I admit I wasn't thrilled to see him.

"What happened?" I asked, stroking the little dog's ears. He nudged my hand when I tried to stop.

"A van hit him." The man was visibly shaken, and his young son distraught.

"What's his name?"

"Buddy."

I went over the pup while the man filled out the standard client information form. Buddy's gums were pale, which could mean shock or pain, or internal bleeding, or chest trauma that restricted oxygen flow. He was panting hard, and still I could not hear air movement through my stethoscope. His belly was tucked, more so than would be explained by his thin condition. I told myself it could be worse. It could be distended, filled with blood.

When I moved my hands over his pelvis, as gently as I could, they met the distinct grinding sensation of bone-on-bone. Actually, it felt like a bag full of bones, but Buddy just turned his mournful eyes to look at me. He never even whimpered.

"He's pretty badly injured," I told the man. A glance at the chart gave me his name: Jim Arcadia. Belatedly, I introduced myself and he told me how it had happened.

"We've only had him a few days. I wanted to get a dog for my son to play with, so I took him down to the pound and they found each other. Buddy was about to get put to sleep that day. I never thought he could get out of our fence."

Apparently the little dog hated being left alone. But Mr. Arcadia was determined he would sleep outside. "We got him partly as a watch dog," he explained.

I nearly burst out laughing. This was the sort of dog who might "watch" a burglar come in, and "watch" him leave again, and if it were in his power he would show the intruder where the valuables were stored, just for a pat on the head.

But I managed to keep a straight face as Mr. Arcadia described his six-foot fence made of vertical wood slats. "I don't see how he got out," he said again. "All I can figure is, he climbed up on the air conditioner and jumped, but that's only two–three feet high, and it's several feet away from the fence!" He shook his head in wonder.

Be that as it may, the dog *had* gotten out, and had dashed into the street and beneath the wheels of a passing van. The driver stopped and rang their doorbell until they woke up. It wasn't his fault. He didn't see the dog until it was too late.

"I'm going to start by taking X-rays of his pelvis," I said. "And his chest, too. I don't like the way he's breathing."

Mr. Arcadia nodded and took his son to wait up front.

Sharon helped with the films. I winced each time I felt the crunch of bone fragments, and by the time we finished I was sweating from empathetic pain. Buddy had whimpered once, when we rolled him onto his back and tried to stretch his legs behind him for the pelvis shot. The worry in his face increased but he didn't resist.

The films were worse than I expected.

The pelvis was bad enough. But given time, and cage rest, that would heal. Even the dislocated hip was straightforward enough. If it wouldn't stay in place, a simple operation to remove the head of the femur would restore function to the joint.

But the chest X-rays made me cringe. Buddy had the worst diaphragmatic hernia I'd ever seen.

"Guess you won't have to confirm this one with barium, huh?" Sharon said half-jokingly. Because sometimes you can't tell.

But every movable organ that should have been in Buddy's abdomen had shoved its way into his chest cavity, tearing a hole in his diaphragm, the flat muscle that normally prevents this from happening.

The diaphragm also accounts for about half the active work of breathing. So he had to move his abdominal wall with exaggerated effort, while intestines and liver and spleen occupied space the lungs needed to expand fully. The only good news was that none of the organs was filling with gas, or appeared strangulated, or "cut off" from their blood supply.

With a heavy heart I carried the films up to show Mr. Arcadia. Diaphragmatic hernias require surgical repair. Even when everything possible is done for them, a high percentage of patients don't make it. But I wanted to try—Buddy had a way of wiggling under my skin and tucking himself into my heart.

I showed Mr. Arcadia the X-rays. I explained all of Buddy's problems. I described the procedures necessary to give him the best chance at a normal life. The only good aspect was that Buddy would never jump another fence, given the damage to his pelvis.

Mr. Arcadia asked what all that work would cost.

I had to tell him he was looking at well over a thousand dollars, and at least a month of cage confinement. If a second operation was needed for the hip, his total bill could easily surpass two thousand.

He looked at his son. He borrowed the phone and called his wife. In the meantime, I called a local practitioner I knew enjoyed challenging surgery, explained the situation, and got a cost estimate of $600–$700 to do the procedure that day.

"We'll have to put him to sleep," Mr. Arcadia told me.

I didn't answer right away. It was what I'd expected. They'd only had the dog a few days, after all. When they granted him a stay of execution at the pound, they certainly never bargained on a thousand-dollar vet bill, let alone a crippled dog. But I felt there was also an element of betrayal. However illogically, when people rescue a dog, they expect gratitude. They know the dog can't understand what is happening. They may be intellectually aware that dogs have no capacity for gratitude. But when little Buddy, who had barely learned his new name, went to such pains to escape that impenetrable fence, it wounded Mr. Arcadia's pride.

He did not want a dog who loved everyone equally. He wanted a dog that was loyal to his family.

So he signed the euthanasia agreement, paid for the emergency fee and the X-rays, and left.

I drew up the injection. Sharon got Buddy out of his cage and carefully placed him on the treatment table. Buddy's expression seemed to say, "I'm sorry I'm so much trouble. I didn't mean to get run over!"

Sharon held off a vein and I slipped the needle in. Blood flowed back into the syringe. In a matter of seconds, he would be dead.

"You know," I said, "we don't repair a lot of diaphragmatic hernias."

"No, that's true."

"I could stabilize him until tonight, and Becky could use the practice, too." Becky had been with us for quite a while, but seemed to miss all the good surgery cases. This one posed a special problem: Since the operation would require opening the dog's chest cavity, he would require artificial means to breathe. We did not own a ventilator at the time, so for the entire duration of the procedure, the tech would have to ventilate the dog by squeezing a rubber bag full of oxygen every ten to fifteen seconds. The surgeon then would have to dodge the lungs, which repeatedly fill and deflate while she is trying to repair the hole in the diaphragm.

"It would be good for her." Sharon was having a hard time with this, too.

Heck, it would be good practice for me, too.

I pulled the needle out. We replaced it with an intravenous catheter and started fluids, antibiotics and painkillers. We made Buddy as comfortable as possible in a cage. He'd be on his own all day, sedated and relatively pain-free. He could die on his own, and if that happened I would have to deal with it.

I must make it clear now that I knew I was technically breaking the law when I failed to put little Buddy to sleep as I had agreed. At the time I rationalized that the form did not state when the injection would be given, and that eventually I would give it, perhaps after surgery. Diaphragmatic hernia repair is one of the more difficult procedures I've ever been called upon to perform, and this little dog presented a golden opportunity.

I also believe, now as I did then, that Mr. Arcadia did not want Buddy dead. He simply did not want Buddy anymore. I have never done such a thing before or since, but for some reason I simply could not kill that pup that morning.

So we left him. It was nearly ten when I got home, and my dog Moby greeted me with his usual enthusiasm. Most of his eagerness was directed toward my clothes, which always carried fascinating scents when I came home from work. Moby had been an only dog for a while, and I imagined he was lonely. I wondered what he would think if a little golden dog came to live with us.

Buddy did fine; in fact, he was much brighter by the time I arrived back at work that evening. We continued the pain medication and antibiotics until midnight, then went to surgery. Becky handled herself perfectly, and Buddy did okay under anesthesia.

Inside, things looked even worse than on film. At first, I couldn't figure out why the abdominal organs seemed so tangled, why they did not slip easily back where they belonged. As I sorted them out, I understood. Buddy had not one but *two* rents in his diaphragm, parallel fissures that left a ribbon of thin muscle between them. Organs had passed into the chest cavity through one tear, then back through the other.

It's like working in a hole. The defect went all the way down to near the dog's aorta. I could feel that main artery throbbing against the back of my hand as I tried to hold the liver out of the way of the suture needle. It was necessary to grasp the edge of the tear with thumb forceps held in my left hand while trying to see around all those organs I had stuffed back into the abdominal cavity. With my right hand I had to keep the liver back and, using an instrument to guide the needle, place a suture through first one, then the other side of the torn muscle.

The flat diaphragm is strong until it is compromised. This strip was shredded at the edges and reluctant to hold a suture. I took large bites and overlapped the margins. It was too wide to remove, it would simply have to hold.

I sutured forever. Becky timed the forced respirations around my stitches, but I had to be absolutely sure I didn't snag the lung with that sharp needle as they leapt repeatedly into the gap. I poked the liver a number of times, but fortunately it is much more forgiving. It was an amazingly unbloody operation, given the amount of damage.

Finally I reached the last suture in the second tear. Before I pulled the gap completely closed I had Becky inflate the lungs and hold while I tied my knot. This helps displace the air that fills the chest cavity and prevents the lungs from inflating afterward. I would still place a chest tube, but Buddy's lungs appeared remarkably healthy, considering what they had endured.

He woke up smoothly. By the next morning he was wagging his tail. Within a few days it was getting hard to keep him in his cage. I started letting him lie at my feet in the office during slow times. Periodically he would get up and put his face in my lap. This little dog who was already on his third home assumed I was his new master.

I had replaced his dislocated hip while he was under the anesthetic, and he now wore his left hind leg in a sling. His pelvis had to hurt like crazy, but he would climb to his feet and hobble after me to go outside and eliminate. He relished every scrap of attention that came his way, and for this reason I think he enjoyed being a patient.

After two weeks I removed the sling that confined his leg. X-rays revealed that the joint had not stayed in place. His pelvis, which should have been nearly square on the films, was deformed into something of a diamond shape. His hind legs would not abduct—they would not move outward beyond straight up and down. This was due to the new shape of his supporting structure.

A friend who does a fair amount of orthopedic surgery came out and removed the head of the femur, leaving him a false joint. He rebounded from that procedure quickly.

In all, he spent nearly a month at the clinic. During that time he was referred to as "the little gold mutt," or "Buddy," or "Lil's dog." I had decided to take him home. The night before, I brought Moby in to see how the two would get along. They did fine.

If I was going to keep him he would need a different name. He was so blond, my friend Joan suggested a Scandinavian name. I thought he was a comical little dog, and wanted to give him a name that reflected his personality. I had a *Far Side* calendar on my desk Joan had given me the previous Christmas, oddball cartoons drawn by Gary Larson before he retired.

Larson. Larson it was.

And so he went home with Moby and me. I felt confident that, with his reconfigured pelvis, he could not jump or climb my fence. I had already ordered him his own name tag, with my phone number and that of the clinic, and bought him a collar. I had picked a time when I had a few days off, so he could get used to his new home while I was around. He followed me everywhere I went.

Then it came time to go back to work. I put Moby and Larson in the backyard, made sure they had plenty of food and water, and left for work.

About nine o'clock, we got a phone call. My lost dog had been found.

Lost? "How did he get out?" I asked. Of course, no one knew. The man who called said he just wandered into his house. He had four dogs of his own, and Larson had apparently been seeking company. I couldn't leave to go get him, so the man grudgingly agreed to keep him overnight. I got directions to his house, and stopped by on my way home the following morning. Larson danced in ecstasy when he saw me. The man was gracious about it—he was a contractor who bought run-down houses, lived in them while fixing them up, then sold them and moved on to the next project.

Once home, I walked the fence in my backyard. It was mostly intact. I reinforced a few loose boards, but decided skinny little Larson had probably slipped between the horizontal slats that were nailed on alternating sides of the fence posts. I went to the hardware store and picked up two bales of chicken wire and spent most of the day stapling it along the inside of my fence. Then I went to work.

The call came earlier this time. Larson had headed straight for the same house at which he had spent the previous night.

Embarrassed, I again arranged to pick him up the next morning. Once again, the little gold dog was thrilled to see me and hopped readily into the cab of the truck. He had already learned to climb between the seats into the space behind them for the ride.

Upon new inspection, I discovered a tunnel under the fence into the yard behind mine. From there, he could slip between the slats and cross the street to the wonderful (from his point of view) house where the back door was left open and someone was home.

I dropped some dog feces into the hole—a trick I'd learned somewhere to discourage digging—and filled it in. I lay bricks along the base of the fence where it intersected the yard in question. I did not get any calls that night about an escaped Larson, and congratulated myself on having solved the problem.

But when I arrived home the next morning, no Larson. I checked the yard—no fresh holes, and the chicken wire remained intact. I stood at the back fence and called his name for several minutes. Finally he came galloping full-bore, his misshapen pelvis giving him a sideways, goofy gait, stopping to slip with practiced skill through the slats of the fence in the yard behind ours. He got to the fence separating the two and stopped. He could not get back in. The fence leaned slightly toward the other yard. I climbed over, lifted him across, then struggled back to my own yard.

I took Larson to work with me the next few nights. He loved it. Moby had to come along, too, of course. He was alternately jealous and solicitous of his new friend. Moby loved getting in the truck but within minutes of arrival wanted to go home. He's a shy dog, not comfortable at the clinic, which was part of the reason I'd gotten him a companion. It was no better this way, as well-disciplined Moby stayed in the office while Larson escaped at every opportunity, to run out front and greet whomever was handy. This was not working.

On my next day off, I let the two dogs outside to play. An hour or so later I let Moby back in. Larson had vanished again. I called his name, with no response. I called the contractor whose house Larson had gone to before. He hadn't seen him. I asked jokingly if he wanted another dog. He didn't.

I called Palm Springs Animal Control to let them know he was out, and took a walk through the neighborhood. No Larson.

Hours later the phone rang. A young boy who lived a block away had found my lost dog. He wanted to know if there was a reward. I tried not to laugh. I did give him a couple of dollars when I picked Larson up. Larson was thrilled to see me. He followed me home without a backward glance. I still wasn't sure how he'd gotten out.

Moby always seemed a bit disappointed when I returned with the little mutt. His energy level was low. After a few minutes of chase and a little muzzle-thrusting play, he was ready for a nap. That's when Larson would go looking for company.

This time I put him outside alone, and watched through the sliding glass door. Larson wandered the yard briefly, then went to a precise spot along the fence and began climbing. It was painful to watch this crippled little dog struggling to balance his weight on the narrow slats of the five-foot-high fence. But he'd obviously had practice, and made the top in seconds, tumbling over in a heap. He bounced back up and headed for the opposite fence.

I called him and he turned around. He'd learned his new name quickly, and cheerfully waited for me to climb over and rescue him. This new game was one he could get into. But it was clear to me I wouldn't be able to restrain him with the current fence.

That night I went out to dinner with a friend. I left the dogs inside. I returned home to a disaster. House plants, sofa cushions, dirt and stuffing were strewn around the living room and ground into the carpet. Moby huddled miserably in the bedroom. Larson greeted me with elation—and very dirty feet.

I was in despair. Once again, this engaging little dog had found himself in the wrong home. He needed constant companionship. I needed self-sufficient pets. I could build a bigger fence—an expense I could not afford—or I could crate him while I was gone. I could take him everywhere I went, or attempt to train him against both his separation anxiety and his gregariousness. None of these felt like a good option. Larson simply needed to belong to someone who was home most of the time. I would never be that person.

Yet, by saving his life I had become responsible for him. I should have euthanized him the morning he was brought in. Now, on the way to the clinic with Larson behind the seat, I realized that's what I would have to do. He didn't fit my life, I couldn't change my lifestyle to accommodate him, and I didn't want to inflict his habits on anyone else. I dropped him off at the clinic, so choked up I could hardly tell Sharon what had happened.

I left him in a run. I went home to clean up the mess and think about what I had done.

Everyone on the emergency clinic staff had gotten to know Larson during his stay. No one could bring herself to administer a euthanasia injection. So for weeks more he languished at the clinic, unable to escape from the run, miserable in solitude. Yet he rarely barked or howled, merely leaning hopefully against the door to his enclosure and following the movements of anyone in sight, hoping for a reprieve. During slow times he came out, lay at the feet of anyone holding still, insisted on following me if I moved. He ignored Red and Tex, and became something of a fixture. He seemed to accept his confinement, but I couldn't miss the hope in his eyes each morning as I left. We were bonded. I had to figure out a solution for him.

The staff put the word out that he was here, and available. A few people came to check him out, families with children, couples with other dogs, but all balked when they heard about his history. No one wanted to take on a problem like this one.

One weekend a retired widower named Ragsdale brought in his very old Pekingese. The dog was on its last legs, emaciated and blind and deaf, creaky with arthritis and barely able to lift its head. The dog hadn't eaten in days, and diarrhea stained his hindquarters. He thought the dog was around sixteen years old.

In such circumstances, people tend to tell me about the tragedies of their lives. Mr. Ragsdale had buried his wife after a long bout with cancer, a son had died of AIDS, and his other children had scattered across the continent like leaves in the wind. For three years the little Peke on the table had been his closest friend, had curled up next to him in bed, had licked the salty tears from his face when loneliness became too much to bear.

But now his friend was dying, and he knew the kindest thing to do was stop the suffering. With tears streaming down his face, he signed the form authorizing euthanasia. He would be going home to an empty house.

Larson, never well-disciplined, had followed me into the room. He approached Mr. Ragsdale, leaned against his leg, and gazed up at him. Larson's stare at once conveyed sympathy and pleaded for affection. Carefully, the man sat down and began rubbing Larson's ears. Over the course of a few minutes, Larson insinuated himself onto the man's lap. He lay on his back, curled into a "C," his mouth hanging open in a grin. He distracted the man while I left with the old dog. Mr. Ragsdale spent several minutes in the room with Larson, the little dog ecstatic in his new role as grief counselor.

It didn't happen right away. After sixteen years, Mr. Ragsdale wasn't quite ready to bring home a new friend. I think many people feel they are somehow betraying the memory of one pet by adopting a new one right away. However, a few days later Sharon called me to the phone. It was Mr. Ragsdale.

"That little dog . . ."

It couldn't have been more perfect. He was home virtually all the time, and could put the dog in his walled, shaded patio if he had to leave for a few hours. Larson adored him, and I'm sure this became mutual within hours of arrival in his new home. I never heard from him again, but I can picture the two of them watching TV, taking long walks of an evening—stopping to chat, perhaps, with dog-loving widows who spot the sweet-tempered mutt and a man in need of friendship.

Most Of My Patients
Are Animals

I've often been asked if I wasn't frightened, being alone all night in the building with one other woman, in a neighborhood not known for its gentle atmosphere. And at times, I had to admit it bothered me. But we locked the door after midnight, sometimes earlier, and didn't open it to anyone who wasn't carrying an animal, preferably someone who had called first.

Which is not to say we didn't get some odd clients late at night. Of course, no one is at their best at this hour, especially when worried enough about a pet to bring it to the vet in the middle of the night. People came in wearing bathrobes, pajamas, nightgowns, grubby sweats with holes in them. They came without makeup, without showering, without combing their hair. I rarely noticed, except peripherally, until I saw them again the next morning. Then they were transformed into lawyers, nurses, office workers—ordinary folk picking up the dog before heading to work for the day.

Still, a few stand out. Like the guy who ran in wearing boxer shorts . . . and nothing else. He'd been in the shower—wet hair still dripping—when his golden retriever had knocked over the empty beer bottle he'd left on the coffee table, broken it and cut an artery. Arteries bleed a lot, and fortunately this one looked much worse than it was. Unfortunately, the guy didn't have his wallet on him, which was understandable at the time, but we never did get paid for saving his dog's life. This was in the days of fairly liberal credit policies. Call me cynical, but today I'd hang on to the dog until he went home and got some money!

And I listened to more sad personal stories than I could ever have imagined. One man whose dog had mammary cancer, which had been neglected too long, accepted the news with a stoical lack of expression. Then he went on to describe in a monotone his wife's recent death after a drawn-out struggle against the same thing. He described massive decubital wounds, the incontinence, and her misery, and I understood that he had been caring for her at home this whole time. The battle had entirely sapped his life savings, leaving him alone and on Social Security. Now I was telling him his dog would die from the same disease. And he couldn't afford even a token effort at saving her.

I heard about miscarriages, divorces, massive injuries, fires, and recent deaths in the family. Sometimes it seemed all the bad fortune in a person's lifetime had been concentrated into a few awful months, culminating in the death of the family pet. Sometimes these stories were told to garner sympathy, in the hopes I would offer to treat the animal at no charge. But mostly people just needed to talk. Maybe the hospital atmosphere struck a chord, and the emotions—grief, helplessness—triggered these memories. Some of them had no one else to tell their stories to. There were nights I had to fight against saying, "Never mind, I'll pay the bill myself"; other times I wanted to scream, "Shut up, I can't stand any more!" I always tried to be patient, but I know that in some cases I succeeded more than others.

Then there was the old man I just think of as "Scars." It must have been around three A.M. when he showed up with his old dog. He was wearing a zip-up coverall, short-sleeved, denim, the kind a lot of repairmen wear over their clothes in the winter, or with nothing underneath in summer. His dog had an acute and life-threatening condition called gastric dilatation-volvulus syndrome, or "torsion" or "GDV" for short. It requires emergency surgery if the dog has any chance at all. The cost is very high, the prognosis guarded even with treatment. The only viable alternative is humane euthanasia.

It can be tough to convince a late-night client of this, especially when the dog is so stoic he's still wagging his tail. Of course, that's when they have the best chance, so I try to talk fast.

Sometimes one glance at a client tells me whether they can afford what their pet needs, but very often my initial impression is absolutely wrong. The later it gets, the less accurate these readings are. So every client hears my full spiel, the long-but-hurried explanation of how the dog's stomach has turned over in its abdomen, is dilated with air and fluid, and won't go back on its own. This leads to shock, as the distended organ cuts off blood flow back to the heart, and blood pools in the hindquarters. The stomach and often the spleen lose their blood supply, and toxic chemicals build up and begin to leak into the system. This leads to more heart problems, and in fact heart failure is the usual cause of death. But there's a tremendous amount of pain and mental distress leading up to that death. The operation to replace the stomach in its normal position and sew it in place has a high rate of success but also a high rate of complications. The total hospital bill is always in the thousands of dollars. If the client cannot afford this, the poor suffering dog should be euthanized immediately.

Imagine explaining that to someone at three A.M., when he just brought his dog in for a stomachache. For "trying to vomit but nothing comes up." Now imagine this is an older gentleman who, let's say, isn't exactly tracking right. The word "operation" triggered a desire to talk.

"I've had operations before," he told me. "See this scar?" He held out a wrinkled forearm. An equally shriveled white ladder ran much of its length. "Left over from the Big One. Shrapnel. Broke both bones in my arm, they had to operate twice."

"But this time, for your dog, I need to—"

"Last year I had a bypass. Triple bypass." And he unzipped his coverall to show me that one. There wasn't anything between the coverall and the scar except sparse gray hair.

Oh, boy, I thought. "Mm, mm," I said. "Listen, about Senator. This is really important, you need to make a decision or it will be too late." Already the dog's gums were losing their pink tinge, becoming cyanotic. He shifted restlessly on the table, his scruffy tail thudding half-heartedly against the countertop. His expression showed concern but not panic. "His heart will give out, and then even a bypass won't help!"

My attempt at humor barely slowed him down. "Then before that, I had to have my appendix out." The zipper came down a little farther and he pointed at a nearly invisible line.

I knew what he was doing. Senator was an old dog, and had been with him since he was a pup. "Scars" did not want to hear what I was telling him. He did not want to tell me to put his old friend to sleep, but the prognosis was lousy and the cost would be too high. I'd encountered this state of denial many times, knew about the combined emotions that caused people to turn the discussion to themselves. In his case there was a hope that it would somehow change my mind, make me tell him something different. Make me say, "Oh, in that case, never mind! My mistake! Just give him these pills and he'll be fine."

Of course, most people don't even realize they're doing it. Most eventually face the fact that I can't choose their pet's illness, I can only diagnose and make recommendations for treatment. Sometimes the options are all lousy.

"My wife died last March," "Scars" was telling me. I wasn't surprised. I'd learned to recognize that certain aloneness. "Senator was her dog." Some people live long enough to lose everything important in their lives, and "Scars" was one. But I couldn't help that, and Senator was going downhill rapidly.

"Do you understand what I'm telling you about Senator?" I asked gently.

He glanced at me, then stared at Senator for a long minute. Then, "I had a hemorrhoid taken out a few years back."

"Don't show me that one!" I said hastily. He'd seemed about to. "Do you have any questions about Senator's condition?"

Another long moment dragged by. He blinked, as if confused now that I'd stopped his display.

"I guess I do," he finally admitted. "Fact is, he hadn't got much time anyhow. I guess I knowed his time was coming. Do I have to stay with him?"

"Not if you don't want to." The graveyard tech had the form ready. "Scars" signed it and followed her to the front desk where he could pay his bill. Once he was out of the room I drew up the injection and put an end to Senator's misery.

But not to his owner's. I never did get to sleep that night.

Macaw Tales

I have always enjoyed working on birds, especially parrots in all their variety. Those intelligent, mischievous faces with the ready beaks that always appear to be smiling . . . even while they chew their way out of their carrying cages. I like their personalities and I enjoy the challenge they present as patients.

Parrots are not like other animals. They do not tell their owners when they are sick. Having evolved as other animals' food, they instinctively hide their symptoms until often it's too late to help them. In the wild, a sick or injured bird is easy prey, so they naturally pretend to be as healthy as possible. Thus the "emergency" sick bird I saw was frequently in the final throes of a chronic illness the owner never even suspected.

Then there are injuries. Birds do find spectacular ways of hurting themselves. They fly into windows, into ceiling fans, into bathtubs full of water. They fall off their perches, sometimes for no discernible reason. They fight with other birds, they tease the dog or escape their cages in the presence of cats. They cut themselves on tiny pieces of toys that they have sharpened with their own beaks. They catch their feet between cage bars and fracture legs.

For some reason the birds with the greatest propensity for major injury are the biggest, most glamorous, and therefore most expensive. I'm talking about the mother of all parrots, the macaws.

The worst I saw was a once-gorgeous scarlet macaw who had recently been moved into an outdoor aviary. The owner, Mr. Jacobs, was proud of his aviary, thinking his birds would be happier outside. It was equipped with a misting system so they wouldn't overheat, and part of it was covered so they could escape the weather in what passes for winter in the desert. He had half a dozen of the huge birds in there, off the patio, a glamorous display to be seen and admired.

But it was surrounded by only one thickness of heavy-gauge wire mesh fencing. The crosshatches left one-inch-square holes between the macaws and the rest of the world. The owner failed to account for wildlife.

Late the second night after the big move outdoors, a raccoon visited the enclosure. Of course, since the fence was bird-proof, the raccoon could not enter the cage itself. But this extraordinary little predator is not so easily deflected. Perhaps it had even been there the previous night, casing the joint, as it were. Or maybe it just got lucky.

Here's what almost certainly happened: The raccoon tried to climb the fence, or jumped at it, which frightened the macaws inside. A bird's natural instinct, when it thinks its life may be threatened, is to fly away. Parrots do not see in the dark, but blind flight has, evolution-wise, resulted in distance from predators, and would certainly be better than no flight at all. When both wings are clipped, these efforts result in an awkward descent to the ground. Being grounded is worse than being isolated on a perch, so the hapless parrot immediately walks to the nearest vertical object—the cage side, for example—and starts to climb.

It uses its beak and feet to climb. The raccoon grabbed one foot in its mouth—or perhaps in its "hands"—and pulled. This resulted in terrified flapping, and the same or another raccoon then managed to snatch a wing. Between the raccoons' pulling and chewing, and the bird's attempt to free itself, both the wing and the leg on one side were horribly mangled.

I saw Mickey the macaw at around three A.M. He was weak with shock and both limbs were beyond salvation. He was not especially tame, so our handling of him only added to his stress.

I said, "He's much too badly traumatized. You can see that. We'll have to put him down."

"I've made up my mind I'll never do that to one of my animals. I want to do everything possible to save him."

"But—" I couldn't believe it. "He can't possibly survive. He's in horrible pain."

"I understand. I hope you'll keep him as comfortable as possible."

"He's lost the wing and the leg on the same side of his body! He'll never be able to get around! And the leg . . . the damage extends too high to amputate. Please, let me put him down!"

But Mr. Jacobs was adamant. The bird was his property, so legally my hands were tied. I agreed to treat the bird overnight if he would transfer it to his vet the following morning. He said he would.

Reluctantly, I began treatment. I started the usual fluids and antibiotics—birds are not so different from mammals when treating for shock. I gave Mickey steroids for shock and pain, a made-up dose of a stronger pain killer, hoping to make him as comfortable as possible until he died on his own, which surely would happen soon. Or if the bird was still alive at eight, at least he would be transferred and out of my hands.

He didn't die.

Mr. Jacobs didn't show up.

I called, got a machine, left a none-too-friendly message. I tube fed the poor bird, gave him more painkillers, and left him in the incubator for the day, expecting to find him dead when I returned that night.

He was still alive. The whole clinic was beginning to stink from rotting tissue. I was angry at myself for trying so hard, but I was furious with Jacobs.

When he called that night I once again asked for permission to euthanize the bird. He again refused. I told him fine, then I would need to take the bird to surgery that night to remove the dead limbs. I made sure he knew the bird was not likely to survive the procedure. He knew. He just didn't want to be responsible for its death. He wanted to know he had done everything he could.

Poor Mickey died almost as soon as he was under anesthesia. Closer inspection of the injuries revealed a deep gash that extended beyond the leg into the muscle of his breast. The wing was torn well into his back. I shed a few tears for this elegant creature, forced to endure a full day of agony while his shredded limbs rotted on his body because of his owner's ignorance and ego and neglect. It would have been kinder to let the raccoons finish what they had started. Or maybe I should have anesthetized him immediately upon his arrival, saving us both all that grief. Good medicine had dictated he be stabilized first; I'm not sure there was a right answer.

But at least Jacobs had spent the day bringing his birds back inside and arranging for a second aviary fence eight inches outside the first. I never treated another bird for him, so I can only assume it worked.

The next raccoon-induced injury I treated wasn't nearly so horrible. It was the same story to start with, except in this case the young, hand-raised blue-and-gold macaw was a beloved pet instead of part of a collection. The owners, Tom and Rick, had believed they were doing their friend a favor building it a lovely outdoor aviary, but had made the same mistake of using only one layer of fence. But this time the raccoon had ripped only one wing, and Bluebell was still in reasonably good shape when she arrived.

My first inclination was to bandage the wing and stabilize her for surgery the following morning. However, she was having no part of that. Four attempts met with instant failure as Bluebell shredded the bandage before I could finish putting it on. She was agitated and distressed, not an ideal surgical candidate at two A.M., but I had no choice.

Sharon and I took her into Treatment and masked her down with isoflurane. Tom stayed and watched. In the interest of speed, I amputated at the site of injury, only clipping off the sharp end of protruding bone instead of cutting it back to remove the contaminated segment. I figured her regular vet could always take out a little more, or take it to the shoulder joint later if needed. I quickly trimmed away shredded skin and sewed the remnants as best I could over the exposed bone. Thank God birds heal fast!

Then I sat on the floor with Bluebell wrapped in a towel to keep her warm and cradled in my lap while she recovered from the anesthesia. I'd given the requisite injections while she was out. Now I chatted with Tom, in a quiet voice aimed at soothing the macaw while she woke. With the fingers of one hand, I stroked her head and neck. A long time passed.

I began to wonder whether Bluebell was going to wake up at

all. Then I felt a foot twitch, ever so slightly. Then nothing. Her head was down, her eyes closed. She didn't move.

I stopped scratching her head and watched. One wise-looking eye slid open, moved from Tom to me and closed again. Bluebell was playing possum.

Altering my tone of voice I said, "Okay, time to wake up!" I unwrapped the towel and was rewarded by feet clutching the fabric. I disentangled them and placed her on the floor of a cage. She immediately stood up and spread her wings—wing—and fell over sideways. Her balance was a mess with one normal and one foreshortened wing. But she was awake and curious and ready to eat.

She never required another operation. I called her regular vet several days later and was told the amputation site was healing beautifully and that Bluebell had lost no time in adjusting to her loss. She was no longer as spectacular when she held her wings out for inspection, but her delightful personality was undampened.

They sent me a picture. She's beautiful.

She only goes outside during the day, and with supervision. And she'll never again need to have her wings trimmed.

Then there was Sam. Six months earlier I'd been plugging along after an unhappy work situation resulted in the departure of our most recent associate veterinarian. It was difficult to manage without someone else—it meant working extra shifts and prevailing on local vets to fill in. The first few months had not been bad, but with the onset of summer and vacations and the wearing thin of my requests, I was having a harder time filling the schedule every month. And then a young veterinarian named Cindy Bacmeister came to my rescue.

Cindy had exceptional diagnostic skills and a strong interest in exotic animal medicine. But, like myself at that stage, she lacked surgical experience.

When one of the hotels brought in a blue-and-gold macaw named Sam whose lacerated right leg they had bandaged too tightly, Cindy was on duty. The original wound had been stitched successfully, but Sam would not leave the sutures alone. So, after discussing the situation with the original vet, the caretaker had bandaged the leg. The result was a loss of circulation that was not noticed for three days, by which time it was too late. The leg was dead. It would have to be amputated.

Sam had once been a pet, and was content with people. Somehow he had ended up at the hotel to be used as a breeder, a task with which he also seemed content. But could he perform with only one foot? Male parrots copulate by standing on the female's back and executing some pretty fancy tail-to-tail maneuvers. It requires superior balance and no small amount of strength.

Even as a pet, his fate as a one-legged macaw was questionable. These are heavy birds, and parrots as a group never lie down. They spend their entire lives standing, flying (in the wild), or perching. They rest their legs, one at a time, by tucking them under their bellies while they sleep.

It was Saturday. The caretaker didn't know what to do. She tentatively authorized the amputation, left the bird in Cindy's care and went to attempt to reach her boss.

Sam was a clown. Though clearly not feeling well with his dead leg, he managed to entertain the staff with his one-word vocabulary: "Hello!" and his insatiable curiosity. Standing at the front of his cage, balanced on his one good foot and dragging the bad one unfeelingly, he greeted everyone who passed. Rocky, my African gray parrot who lived in Treatment, was enchanted.

Because the leg was now a dangling piece of dead tissue, and was beginning to rot, Cindy felt that time was of the essence. When she didn't hear from the caretaker for several hours, and was unsuccessful in reaching her, she decided to proceed with the amputation. She was nearly through when the call came. The higher-ups had decided to cut their losses. The caretaker requested that Cindy euthanize Sam.

It's hard to explain the bond that forms between a veterinarian and a patient. By this time Cindy felt she was committed to the bird. But when Rebecca told her Sam had stopped breathing, she assumed it was an anesthetic complication and decided to finish the operation for the practice.

But Sam wasn't dead. Birds, with their odd respiratory system, can actually breathe passively, and I've been fooled more than once into thinking one was in trouble while on gas. When Cindy finished her work she checked his heart, and it was beating fine. In fact, since he'd been taken off the gas at the first sign of trouble, he was now waking up.

"Oh, boy. Now what do I do?" Cindy asked her patient.

Sam had no answer. Cindy called me and explained the situation.

We discussed it and I said, "I think you need to call them and get permission to adopt the bird. Just tell them exactly what happened. If they insist on putting it down, we really don't have a choice."

"I think they just wanted to not spend the money. Can I get them to do a retroactive donation?"

"I don't see why not. But then, someone has to keep him. Are you willing to do that?"

She hesitated. Cindy was already applying for residencies. She would be going back to school, taking her dog and her rabbit. She would be working long hours. Macaws are highly social birds. They need frequent attention. The demands of a residency were not compatible with single-bird ownership. "I wouldn't inflict my lifestyle on another animal," she finally said.

"Well, there won't be a huge market for one-legged macaws. But we can keep him at the clinic for a while and see what happens."

I worked the next day and watched Sam learn to balance on one leg. He'd been doing it anyway, but now he lacked even the stabilizing dead post the missing limb had been. He would grip the side of the cage with his beak and pull himself up. Then he would spread his wings for balance, leaning slightly to the left. By the end of the day he had learned to stand without support.

Unused to the pelleted diet Rocky unwittingly shared with him, Sam at first refused to eat. We offered him fruits and corn, which he nibbled at. Normally he would have held a piece of fruit, or a wheel of corncob, in one foot while pulling off bites with his beak. The loss of that ability was traumatic for him. Add to that the stress of being removed from familiar environs, and losing his mate. Sam was suffering from an avian version of depression.

Yet he needed calories. Even more so now than usual, while his body recovered from the double whammy of injury and surgery. So for a day or two we tube fed him a formula designed for hand-rearing baby parrots.

Fortunately, he was a resilient bird. He was already making friends with the staff, and Cindy stopped in to check on him that evening. By Tuesday he was eating on his own, even sampling the pellets. During a quiet period, I took him into the office and placed him on my lap. Seemingly grateful, he rested his weight on his keel and used his only foot to scratch his face and the back of his head. He preened a little, enjoyed a good scratch from me, then went to sleep. It was the first of many such episodes.

The fact that Sam could scratch himself while on my lap, but not while in his cage, bothered me. He couldn't balance on his chest on a flat surface. We tried giving him towels to lie on, but he just got his toenails tangled in them. We did not have an actual bird cage for him, nor was there room for one, so he'd been making do with a perch in a standard dog cage. His tail feathers were broken and dirty despite the techs' efforts to clean him.

He enjoyed getting out. His favorite place, other than a lap, was the wet table—a sort of raised shallow bathtub with a grate over it. Rocky's cage was nearby, and the two formed a loose bond. Rocky took to standing on one foot whenever Sam was nearby. But he became aggressively jealous whenever one of the staff paid too much attention to Sam and not enough to Rocky.

Most of a week went by. Sam stayed at the clinic. We still didn't know what to do with him.

Then Nancy Carlson worked a Friday night. She'd always been drawn to birds, though not as patients. When she heard Sam's story she immediately offered to adopt him.

He stayed at the clinic for most of a month. The sutures came out, and he learned to get around on one leg. Placed on the vinyl floor, he would lean forward so his weight rested on his beak, and hop rapidly, easily outdistancing Rocky on his two good legs. He thrived on the pellets he had earlier disdained. He learned to eat fruit by pushing it into a corner of his food dish, though corn on the cob remained a problem.

Nancy took him to work with her. For two years or more he lived in a cage in the corner of the clinic where she worked for a mostly absentee owner. He frequently escaped from his cage and came hopping into the exam room where Nancy was ensconced with a client. He had rope perches and a grate in one corner of his cage where he could lie down. He had a regular schedule and plenty of entertainment. He could have stayed indefinitely had he not been so fond of screaming.

A big parrot can approach a chain saw in decibels. And Sam had grown cocky and demanding, wanting Nancy's constant attention. This is not conducive to good client relations or to a healing environment. Nancy finally took him home. But she worked long hours and he spent most of his time there alone.

Like many birds deprived of companionship, Sam turned his frustration on himself. He began pulling out his own feathers. When Nancy came home, his screaming was worse then ever. Another couple of years went by, Sam growing bald and miserable. Nancy had long considered finding him a new home, one with other birds, with an owner who spent more time at home. He was a special-needs pet, but there were offers. Still, Nancy demurred.

Meanwhile, one of her technicians, Lisa, had acquired a couple of smaller parrots. She became active in the local bird club and dreamed of filling her house with the noisy imps. When a stray blue-and-gold macaw flew into a local country club, Lisa was offered the chance to adopt it. This was a sleek, tame, and apparently healthy blue and gold macaw that had simply flown in and landed on a low wall at the home of one of Nancy's clients. She and Lisa bonded immediately. And no one ever showed up in response to the "found bird" ads she placed.

It seemed only natural that Sam should move in, too. So that's what happened. It was love at first sight, and the newcomer happened to be female. Sam is doing his best to copulate with only one leg. Odds are the pair will never produce young, but that's fine with Lisa. Despite an occasional scream, the two are happy with each other. Sam's feathers have grown back in. His new mate does not seem to mind his handicap.

But Lisa had to get a new bird. Neither Sam nor his new lover have time for her now. She was lucky enough to win the grand prize at the bird club's annual raffle—a hand-fed baby blue-and-gold macaw.

Never
Too Old

"They're sure it's a reaction to the shot he had for his arthritis three days ago," said the voice on the phone. Kathy Ross, who worked for Dr. Vicki Robertson, another veterinarian in town, was calling on behalf of her neighbors. They were clients of her employer. "But I just don't think so."

"He was fine until tonight?"

"Yeah, and he looks pretty bad right now."

"What's he doing?"

"He keeps trying to throw up and nothing comes out."

"Is his abdomen distended?"

"Hm. Maybe. I think so. Yeah, it is."

"They need to bring him in right away. It's got nothing to do with the shot. It sounds like his stomach."

Champ was a fifteen-year-old German shepherd, scrawny and arthritic and a bit ragged-looking. According to Kathy, it had taken her boss a couple of years to persuade the Bronsons to let her treat his arthritis at all, and that treatment had consisted not of the newer chondroprotective agents but of a single injection of a corticosteroid.

Tonight I could virtually diagnose his problem from across the room. His stomach had twisted and was filling with gas. He had gastric dilatation-volvulus syndrome, GDV for short.

"Stomach," for our purposes, refers not to the space below the chest, but to a specific organ. It looks very much as depicted in those antacid commercials—a little like the drainpipe beneath your sink. It is the chamber where food is stored, mixed with fluid and bile and acid. Chemical bonds begin breaking down in this first stage of the digestive process. It is really a wide spot in the digestive tube, beginning with the esophagus and moving on to the first part of the small intestine.

When the stomach twists, food and fluid cannot escape. Air is swallowed as the dog becomes increasingly anxious, and there it stays. Enough air causes severe distension, which is the main source of the pain these dogs experience. Imagine Thanksgiving dinner. Then imagine sucking on an air hose afterward.

This is a medical condition we learned to fear in school, and which I had dreaded for years after graduation. But I'd finally grown confident in its diagnosis and management. I almost look forward to them now. It practically always happens at night, and is thus the purview of the emergency clinician.

Sharon and I took a quick X-ray of Champ's abdomen to confirm the diagnosis, and I showed it to the Bronsons. They were ordinary middle-aged folk. I'd just met them. I couldn't tell how they would react to the news.

"He'll need immediate surgery to correct the problem," I explained. "Though first we need to treat him for shock and run an electrocardiogram. One of the things that kills these dogs is heart arrhythmias. Then we'll decompress the stomach, anesthetize him and pump it out, then we go to surgery to put it back where it belongs and sew it in place so this can't happen again. A lot can go wrong. He'd be at risk for several days after the procedure. That's assuming he makes it through and wakes up afterward." I've learned bluntness is the best approach in these cases, and there isn't a lot of time for discussion.

They were remarkably calm. "What will happen if we don't have the operation?"

"It's a painful, frightening way to die. I hope, if you can't afford the surgery, you'd let me put him to sleep so he won't have to go through that."

They weren't quite ready to make up their minds. I got IV supplies out so we'd be ready in case they decided to go for it. But I'd been prejudiced by the history. They had refused to treat his painful, nearly crippling arthritis for so long, then eschewed the better drugs in favor of the cheaper one. I doubted they'd be inclined to spend in the neighborhood of two thousand dollars in the face of his age and the questionable outcome of what I was proposing.

"He's so old," Mrs. Bronson said.

"And his arthritis has been so bad. The shot helped, but that's temporary, right?"

I shrugged. They'd already covered those options with their regular vet. "Old age isn't a disease," I said. "But it does complicate things."

They exchanged sorrowful glances. "I think we should put him to sleep. Don't you?" she said so quietly I could barely hear.

Staring at the floor where his dog lay, Mr. Bronson nodded his head. I handed them a box of Kleenex and Sharon headed up front to get the form authorizing me to put the animal down. I got out a 12-cc syringe and the bottle of euthanasia solution, and began drawing up the dose. Sharon returned, filled in the form, and handed it to Mrs. Bronson to sign. As is so often the case, the wife seemed stronger, more able to affix her signature where required.

She took the proffered pen and began to write her name.

Then she stopped.

"I think we should at least give him a chance. Don't you?" She said it in exactly the same tone she had used moments earlier when she'd said just the opposite.

Her husband looked up, hope dawning. "Yes. Yes, I think we should give him a chance."

Both pairs of eyes turned toward me. "Do the operation. Please, Doctor."

Just like that, we swung into full-speed-ahead mode. A catheter went into Champ's vein, fluids ran as fast as they could. Sharon set up the OR while Jane wrote up a cost estimate. I pulled blood and shaved a spot on Champ's side and thrust three or four large-bore needles directly into his stomach to relieve the pressure from the severe gas distension. Despite the dog's attempts to vomit or belch, the contents were trapped in his stomach much like in a balloon with the neck twisted. As foul air escaped, his belly visibly shrank and he appeared to lie more comfortably.

But the torsion also interfered with blood flow, both to the stomach itself and to the spleen closely attached to it, as well as with the blood returning from the hindquarters to the heart. Champ's ancient circulatory system was not well-equipped to handle such insults.

By now the estimate was signed and the OR ready. Sharon helped me lift Champ onto the wet table and hook up the ECG. The tracing was remarkably steady. The blood work I'd started showed no abnormalities serious enough to change our course. I induced anesthesia with a combination of Valium and a narcotic, slipped an endotracheal tube down his throat, and hooked him up to oxygen and isoflurane. Using gentle force, we pushed a wide semirigid plastic tube through the esophagus into his stomach, its arrival announced by a rush of more sour gas, then his sodden dinner and a gallon or so of the water he'd drunk either before this started or once the symptoms began.

Nearly ninety minutes had passed since the dog's arrival. Given everything that had transpired, that wasn't bad.

By the time I opened his abdomen, the flaccid, empty stomach had flopped nearly into a normal position. I've seen that often enough not to be fooled. The spleen, still twisted, was a ticking time bomb. I clamped its vessels without untwisting it—the toxins that had built up while blood flow was cut off could irreversibly affect the heart if allowed back into circulation. It was a simple matter to ligate and cut those large vessels. I dropped the spleen into the sink with a sound like a wet towel.

There is a ligament—nothing more than a band of strong connective tissue—that normally holds the right side of the stomach against the liver. In Champ's case it was long gone. This is the usual finding in GDV. It happens in certain deep-chested dogs, especially those who eat only once daily, or drink large quantities of water, or habitually run or play or roll over with a full stomach. Over time, the ligament stretches under the weight of the overburdened stomach, and activity causes the stomach to move within the abdomen. Eventually the stomach moves the tiniest bit too far, and comes down on the wrong side. Once emptied it may very well slosh back into place. But it will twist again if left untreated.

But the organ was in good shape. I examined it closely, looking for the telltale dark, dull areas that indicate a too-long lack of blood flow. There were none. So far things were looking promising.

So I created a half-thickness flap from the stomach wall and dragged it beneath a rib, sewing it back in place on the other side. The two layers would heal together, creating a scar much stronger than the original ligament. If it survived two weeks after surgery, the bond would be virtually unbreakable.

That done, I closed him up: two layers of dissolving sutures, one in the muscle of his belly and another beneath the skin. Sharon turned off the gas and he breathed pure oxygen while I stapled his skin.

The ECG indicated no ill effects to his heart. We moved him to a blanket in a run and he began waking from the drugs. The Bronsons, who had waited while we worked, came to say good night, then went home. It was after three A.M., and they would have to return in a few hours to transfer him back to Dr. Robertson.

By eight o'clock, Champ had made no attempt to get up. He was awake, and had rolled onto his chest a few times, but that was it. We hefted him onto the stretcher and carried him to the Bronsons' small motor home. I called Dr. Robertson and told her Champ was on his way. I went home to sleep. I wasn't sure what to expect over the course of the day.

That evening he walked back in, if a bit unsteadily.

The next morning he jumped up, wagging his tail when he spotted his owners. At Dr. Robertson's the second day he began to take food and water. She sent him home that night.

A couple of days later I called to see how Champ was doing. Mrs. Bronson came to the phone. "It's the strangest thing," she said. "Would the operation help his arthritis?"

I'd been asked weirder questions. "No reason it should," I answered.

"Well, he's been jumping in and out of the motor home like a puppy!"

"Try not to let him do that for another week or so, okay? He's got a lot of stitches that need to heal."

"Well, I'll try." From her mirthful tone I doubted it. "But we were just talking about it. As soon as this is over, we're going to ask Dr. Robertson about those other treatments. He's like a new dog! We should have had the operation done years ago!"

CAT Scan
For A Dog

Buster had a seizure one night.

Not so unusual. We saw a lot of dogs for seizures. Different things cause them—sometimes we can figure it out, most times we can't. We control the seizures with phenobarbital and Valium, sometimes dexamethasone or glucose or antibiotics, depending on the cause or suspected cause. If nothing shows up on the lab work we treat the symptoms. It's all we can do. If that doesn't work the usual options are euthanasia or referral to a specialty center, where advanced diagnostics are routine.

By far the most common cause of seizures in young dogs is idiopathic epilepsy. "Idiopathic" means we aren't sure what causes it. "Epilepsy" simply refers to seizure disorder. In older dogs, if they haven't been exposed to poisons, the likely etiology is a tumor.

Buster was eleven. That's calendar years, not "dog" years. And he'd never had a seizure before.

"I love this dog," Travis, his owner, told me.

Buster didn't move. Buster was still sedated from the drugs Mindy Byers had used to keep him quiet enough to transfer for the weekend. Mindy was one of my favorite referring veterinarians. Her workups were always thorough and she wasn't afraid to ask someone else's opinion. She'd gotten Buster as a transfer from us that morning, already sedated but still able to walk.

Travis's girlfriend, Tiffie, stood by with tears in her eyes. "I'm so sorry, Trav," she said. Then, to me, "I haven't known him as long as Trav, but he's a great dog. We don't want him to suffer." The tears, somehow, remained poised on her lower eyelids, which were blue.

"Trav" shot her a disbelieving glance. "We want to do everything possible to help him," he said to me while looking at her.

Oh, boy. "Has Dr. Byers talked to you about taking him down to Los Angeles for a neurological workup?"

Tiffie said, "We can't afford that."

Trav said, "I can't afford that." He glanced irritably at Tiffie. "I don't have time, either."

I said, "With every seizure his prognosis gets worse. It would not be wrong to put him to sleep now."

"I know that, but I want to give him every chance," Travis said.

"We don't want him to suffer," Tiffie insisted.

"Tiffie, will you stop saying that? It's my money!"

"All I'm trying to say is, I don't think you should prolong the inevitable."

I already didn't like Tiffie, but she had a point.

Travis looked at me. "Do you think he's in pain, Doctor?"

The all-important question, but largely irrelevant for Buster. "I can honestly tell you no. I don't think he feels anything at this moment."

"There!" He turned to his girlfriend, who was glaring at me through her moussed bangs.

"But that doesn't mean he's comfortable," I pointed out, increasingly uncomfortable with the way the discussion was going. "He's living in a drug-induced coma right now, and it's hard to say exactly what he feels."

"Coma!" Tiffie seized the word. "See, Trav? He's in a coma!"

"That's because of the drugs! Don't you listen?" To me: "When the drugs wear off will he be in pain?"

Why do people latch onto pain? "We can treat pain," I hedged. "But I'm not sure we can let the drugs wear off. He'll just have more seizures."

"Just say maybe he got into something. You know, poison. How long till it wears off?"

Buster's legs began paddling, pantomiming swimming. It was hard to know if this was medication wearing off or the onset of another fit.

"That depends on the poison. Do you think he got into something?" And if so, why hadn't he mentioned it until now? He must have been asked at least three times. Maybe that's where the idea came from.

"It's the only thing I can think of that might explain his symptoms."

I blinked. Mindy, on the phone, told me she'd been over the possibilities with him. Even if he'd been too dazed and tired the night before to understand anything that was said to him, he should have understood by now that the odds of Buster ever going home were akin to his softball team winning the World Series. "As we've discussed, Buster almost certainly has a fast-growing tumor inside his skull," I explained again. "That's why we want to send you to LA. A CAT scan might show the tumor, and tell us whether it's operable, or might respond to radiation." I had, only a month before, sent a ten-year-old schnauzer down while her seizures were still infrequent. She'd had a CAT scan followed by radiation treatment. Her prognosis was good. But even if they took Buster immediately, I didn't think he had the same chance. The seizures were too severe and more or less constant when he wasn't medicated. "Without that, we're shooting in the dark. He can't live like this much longer."

As if on cue, he started another seizure. The previous slow, regular paddling evolved into a stiffening of all four legs, then the lips curled back and he chewed air, saliva turning to foam and coating his lips.

"Ohmigod, he's got rabies, doesn't he?" Tiffie stepped back.

If only it were so easy. "No, saliva does that when it's mixed with air." Sharon had the stretcher ready and together we moved the seizuring dog onto it and into the back room. I gave him another cc of Valium and he relaxed.

"Okay, I'm going to start blasting him with steroids tonight in hopes of shrinking the swelling. The other drugs aren't holding him, and he's getting an awful lot of them."

"Do whatever you can, Doctor," Travis told me solemnly.

Tiffie rolled her eyes, arms crossed over her chest.

The dog had become some sort of symbolic line between these two, and it frustrated me. He could go on like this for days, maybe weeks. We could drip nutrients into his IV line while he seizured and slept until his already thin body wasted to bones and bedsores. It was just the sort of high-maintenance case that robbed the staff of morale, because after the second day they knew we were faking it. That the animal wasn't getting better. They were working on a corpse.

But Travis insisted we continue, and Buster was his dog. Buster might not be suffering, but that was only because he was unconscious. I tried steroids to no apparent avail. I repeated the blood work, all frustratingly normal. I even gave plasma, then dextran, and would have used Hetastarch had it been available to us at the time, all in hopes of reducing what I supposed was increased pressure on the dog's brain. He had a few minutes of relatively normal awareness, and would recognize and respond to his owner by wagging his tail. During these brief periods both of us—Travis and I—would convince ourselves the dog was really improving. Then he'd start twitching, his lips would pull back in that pseudo-grin, and he'd be off to wherever dogs go when their bodies thrash in the throes of a grand mal seizure.

It was one of the times when I'd given him a heavy dose of Valium followed by the second injection of phenobarb in as many hours, when it occurred to me to do a cerebrospinal tap. I hadn't planned on it, since the procedure requires general anesthesia in dogs. If they move at the wrong instant, it could be disastrous. But, though the drugs might not have been the ones I would have chosen, this dog was as anesthetized as he was likely to get.

The other potential problem is, in the case of severely elevated pressure, a spinal needle inserted in the soft spot just below the skull can result in a sudden release of pressure and catastrophic brain injury. But I couldn't help thinking that if his pressure was elevated, something I'd done would have helped by now, at least a little.

I shaved him, surgically prepped him, and had my sample of fluid in minutes. I'd only performed a few of these since graduating, and they had all been as anticlimactic as this one. I psyched myself about all the possible things that could go wrong, then did it, got it done, all in less than a minute.

His pressure did not appear to be elevated. The fluid was disappointingly clear. I realized I'd been half-hoping for something dramatic I could show Travis—blood or pus, anything that would convince him either to let Buster go or take him to a bigger facility. A neurologist, that's what he needed. Someone with a lot more letters after his name than I had.

I sent the clear sample over to the human hospital for analysis. That's where the idea came from.

I'd been attending rounds at one of the hospitals for over a year, and had come to know people in several departments, including Radiology, where the CT scanner lived. I got on the phone with Radiology on Monday morning, and we made arrangements to bring Buster in after hours on Tuesday. I contacted the veterinary radiologist at the referral hospital to which I'd tried to send Buster to get some specifics regarding patient preparation. I was glad I did, as there was more to this than I'd thought. Patient positioning is crucial; the amount of venous contrast dye required was more than we had on hand. I set about borrowing more.

The plan was to smuggle Buster in through the department's back door. I would maintain absolute general anesthesia during the procedure itself using Propofol, a new injectable anesthetic not yet approved for dogs but the best available for the circumstances. I would inject the contrast into his vein and leave the room, and the scan would begin.

In a way just making the plan was a mistake. I'd apprised Travis and Tiffie of what I was doing from the idea's inception. It gave Travis something to strive for, a reason to keep Buster alive, if that word really describes what Buster was. But without it, we would have been left hoping the case would end on its own. The CT date presented a deadline of sorts.

I will not mention the name of the hospital here, but I will say it was not the only time I took an animal in after hours for a procedure, or procured the assistance of medical doctors for a complicated case. I don't think anything we did was illegal, but the reason we chose not to notify the media at the time was fear of patient perceptions. In an era when doctors are being hammered from all directions, it's tragic to see them afraid to publicize a good deed because it might be twisted around by people who illogically fear contamination or some sort of technomorphing alien beams that would cause a machine to become harmful after being used on a dog. Actually, I'm not sure exactly what they were afraid of, but the decision was made not to seek publicity.

As an aside, there is still in existence, as far as I know, a CT scanner at a veterinary school which has been modified to accommodate horses. Unlike the original equipment, this table can support the tremendous weight involved. Normal CT tables are rated, I believe, up to 400 pounds. This lets out a certain portion of our population. As a result, certain very large human patients have been quietly shipped to this veterinary school for years to obtain their specialized procedures. It's nice that we can give back now and then.

At any rate, Tuesday dawned hot and sunny, hardly a surprise in the desert. Buster spent another stuporous day at Desert Animal Hospital. Shortly after six P.M., the Pet Taxi pulled up at the back door of a certain radiology department and unloaded a figure on a stretcher, mostly covered with a white sheet. Travis, Mindy, and I, and even Tiffie, arrived in separate cars.

We moved Buster into a big white room. All that seizuring had dislodged quite a few catheters, and somehow the latest one, which I'd thought was securely anchored, had kinked during the latest transfer. Neither I nor Mindy had brought any more catheters, so I would be required to locate a new vein for both the Propofol, which will not work at all by any other route, and the contrast, which had to go IV in order to reach the brain. After both injections we had a window of only a few minutes before the body excreted the dye.

The procedure was not an overwhelming success. But we got our pictures. Trouble was, none of us knew how to read them.

"Is this an asymmetry?" I asked one of the two radiologists who had stayed to perform the scan.

"I can't tell. Are dogs' skulls always that thick?"

I told him I thought they were. The size of the brain in question was astonishingly small. I mean, I'd seen canine CT scans before—they weren't rare, even then—but I'd never *studied* them. Now, after all the trouble we'd gone to, we had our pictures, and none of us knew how to interpret them.

Buster returned to the emergency clinic. It was my night off, and I went home to sleep. The following day we shipped the films to the radiologist in LA. He graciously read them and barely criticized our technique. He said he thought the dog had a brain tumor.

But by then, things had resolved on their own. Buster's seizures, which had seemed to level off since Sunday morning, suddenly worsened. By mid-Wednesday, they were virtually constant, and refractory to even the highest doses of phenobarbital. Travis went in during his lunch break to say good-bye. As seems to happen so often at the end, Buster lifted his head and looked his master in the eye. But instead of second-guessing his own decision, Travis nodded to Mindy to go ahead with the injection.

Buster died before the diagnosis—brain tumor—came back. The verdict was no surprise to anyone who'd been involved in the case. But somehow, knowing we were willing to go to such lengths on the chance of helping his pet helped a grieving dog owner accept reality.

Travis was finally able to let Buster go.

A Family Cat

Her name was Snowball. She was neither the first nor the last Snowball I ever treated, and she was certainly not the whitest. In fact, this Snowball was a black-and-white shorthair. She lay on her side on the exam table, not even twitching her tail. Her ribs protruded lankly with each breath. There was not a mark on her anywhere.

"She's only two. We got her last year when our first Snowball died," Mr. Lopez, the man who had brought her, explained almost apologetically.

I had finished examining the cat, and was frankly perplexed. "Has she had her shots every year?"

She had. That helped rule out a lot of possibilities, diseases that didn't fit the cat's appearance anyway. "How long has she been like this?"

"Like this? Just today. But we noticed she didn't act right since last Friday." This was Tuesday.

So the onset had been somewhat gradual. "Does she go outside?"

"Yes. We can't seem to stop her." He glanced with the first sign of humor at his two boys, probably six and eight. Clean and neatly dressed, they stood behind the table, gazing solemnly at me. The enormous dark brown eyes held a normal concern: This was, after all, a doctor's office. A place where shots were given. They were not too young, however, to understand that Snowball was very sick.

And she was. She was underweight, but not severely so. She was profoundly dehydrated. But her heart sounded fine and her temperature was normal. Her eyes were dull but undamaged,

155

and focusing pretty well given how apathetic she was to everything around her. The gums were a normal pink, if horribly dry, and even her teeth looked healthy. I simply could not find anything specific to target as a cause for her symptoms. "Have you seen her vomit? Any diarrhea? Coughing or sneezing? *Anything?*"

Three heads shook from side to side.

"Okay, I'll need to start by taking some blood to test her liver and kidneys and her immune system. The most important thing is to get an IV line started, so we can get some fluids into her. That alone is bound to make her feel better. . . ."

I trailed off. Mr. Lopez was shaking his head sadly, looking down at the walker upon which he leaned. He was a young man, in his early thirties. His physical hesitancy had barely registered on me until this moment. "I can't work now. We can't afford all that." He was clearly ashamed to have to admit this, either to me or in front of his children.

I glanced at the kids. A single, silent tear escaped the older boy's eye and ran unchecked down his face.

I looked back at the cat, clearly hours from death if I didn't do something to help her, and do it soon. And of course I still didn't know if there was anything I *could* do.

But somehow she just didn't look like a terminal cat. Her breath did not stink like it should with kidney failure or diabetes. Her body temperature had not fallen into the subnormal range, so common in really sick cats as their systems either give up the fight, or slow the metabolic rate in a last-ditch attempt to prolong life. Her gums were not the white of severe anemia, and I could feel no cancerous mass in her belly. No mucus clogged her nostrils, no ulcers pocked her tongue—it was unlikely that a virus had laid her low.

If I did nothing, she would die. If I did everything, she still might die. But if I could not reach a compromise, Mr. Lopez would ask me to put her to sleep. And then we would both have to face those eerily silent children who felt their father's shame at not being able to save their pet.

This can be a critical situation for kids. They may not clearly understand the difference between the animal and themselves. They had lost one cat the year before; now this Snowball was sick and they knew—could tell, the way children can—that they were about to lose this one. They hadn't said a word, but they knew.

I'd been there before. I have euthanized pets belonging to children. Sometimes I sent the kids with Sharon or Becky to visit Rocky the dancing parrot while I spoke to their parents about the situation. I have allowed them to sign the form and take their children home, enacting a fiction that Fluffy would be living with us now. I have let other parents go to the shelter and select a new kitten that resembled the old one so the children would never know. I have tolerated screaming accusations because I would not treat an animal at no charge, a puppy who had never had a vaccination in its life and had been left in the back yard for days while flies crawled on the food it was too sick to eat.

As a rule I try not to get involved in the fantasies people enact with their children when they are too poor or too ignorant to care for the pets they brought home "for the children." Sometimes this is horribly difficult. Other times I admit that my anger has overshadowed my compassion for the animal unfortunate enough to wind up with such people. It's easy to get jaded after the fourth such case in four days.

But these kids, this man, were different. Clearly educated, he had met some accident that landed him at a young age—my age, approximately—behind this walker. Perhaps their mother was at work now, or maybe he made the effort alone, but the kids were astonishingly well-behaved. Their clothing was old and worn, perhaps handed down or purchased at thrift shops, or left over from better times, but it was clean and so were they.

Snowball had been given good basic care—she was spayed and vaccinated and had obviously been well-fed until she got sick. I could forgive the denial that caused them to wait until the last minute to present her for care. And I knew the resignation in their eyes, the acceptance of the limitations imposed by their unaccustomed poverty.

Besides, I was curious as hell about what was wrong with that cat.

"I'll tell you what. Can you afford a hundred dollars?" The emergency fee was nearly half that already.

He hesitated, then nodded. "Can we do it over time?"

Normally, with an amount that small—an amount I knew

would not begin to cover the actual fees involved—I would have said no. I was an employee. It wasn't my money to give away. But as long as the clinic showed a profit, the board would not question a rare case of compassionate care. The key word here is rare. Voluntary is nice, too. I don't mind occasionally donating services, but I hate being cheated out of them. And if this cat died I felt it was unlikely we would be paid even for the small amount involved. The owner didn't know that yet, but I'd seen it too many times. When the bill comes due and the pet is gone, too many other things come first.

Still, by now I was committed—mentally if not financially. "Okay, leave her with me, and I'll get some fluids into her and start her on antibiotics, then we'll see how she does. Maybe if I just treat the symptoms she's got enough strength to bounce back. But I can't guarantee anything."

The gratitude in his eyes was painful. They thanked me and left the cat.

I had planned to give some electrolyte solution under the skin, an antibiotic injection, and monitor the cat overnight. But we had a new tech in training, so I asked her to put an IV in with Sharon's help. Intravenous solutions enter the circulation faster. And a profoundly injured system like Snowball's can't always be counted on to absorb them subcutaneously.

The cat responded rapidly to rehydration. Within hours she was up on weak legs, beginning to explore her cage. Offers of first water, then food, were consistently declined, so I knew she would not be going home that morning. Since we'd long since used up the hundred dollars, I knew no daytime veterinary clinic wanted the transfer. So she stayed.

By that evening she had begun to vomit. She was alert, mobile, very responsive, but there was no way she could be removed from the IV. I suspected she had been vomiting before, unnoticed, and the primary problem lay in her intestinal tract.

By now I was angry at myself for taking the case on. The cat had indeed improved, so my hunch had been right. But now she was dependent on the IV, and she was my responsibility until I discovered and relieved the underlying problem. All further work would need to be done either at no cost or after exhaustive discussion. And I was sure that discussion would lead to euthanasia. I sighed and drew some blood from the cat.

A few tests confirmed there was no real problem in the cat's major organs. X-rays of her abdomen revealed a small intestine puckered like a string of beads.

"She's got a linear foreign body," I told Becky.

"Cool," she said. "Surgery?"

I had to smile. I had learned to truly enjoy these operations, and so by now had the techs. And at least it was a quiet night.

I quickly telephoned Mr. Lopez and told him I needed to take Snowball to surgery. She'd swallowed a string or something, and it was caught in her small intestine. If I didn't go in and remove it, it would cut through the gut and she'd die of peritonitis. He understood that the operation was necessary. He agreed, and since we would not have a signed release I had him tell Becky as well. No discussion took place as to cost, again because I was committed to the cat.

So we anesthetized Snowball and prepared her belly. The double thickness of sewing thread twined through her gut all the way to the colon, or large intestine. I started near the junction between the stomach and small intestine, making a stab incision into the gut, pulling a tiny length of thread out and cutting it, attaching a hemostat to the long end so I'd have something to tug on to identify other segments. I'd done this procedure before, and usually a sharp tug on the "short" end results in the removal of a piece of the thread. In this case it felt as if it was caught on something. I decided to leave it, finish the rest of the operation, and come back to it.

It took four incisions. Here's how it goes: I followed the gut down several inches, made an incision and pulled a length of thread out, then cut it short, leaving a clamp attached so the new end was not lost. Then I moved farther down the gut, made a new incision and repeated the whole thing. Then I went back and sewed up the previous hole. All the time it was very important to keep the parts of the intestine with open incisions outside the cat's abdomen, because the fluid leaking out was contaminated with digestive enzymes and bacteria, and would lead to peritonitis if much of it got into the belly. The farther down, the higher the concentration of bacteria and the greater the risk of infection—which is why I started near the stomach. With its strongly acid environment, the stomach is almost sterile. The irritating juices wipe off easily, allowing the surgeon to continue without changing gloves at every turn.

Finally, the only thread remaining was a small piece in the large intestine. I would leave that and let it pass on its own, rather than pull it into my incision (because the colon is the dirtiest place in the body). I closed the final incision carefully, and Becky poured warmed sterile saline over the area to clean it off. I slipped the last of the intestine back into Snowball's abdomen and threw away the contaminated paper drape the intestine had been resting on, then changed into new, sterile gloves. It was time to figure out where this thing was stuck.

Where bodies are concerned, it is generally a bad idea to force anything. I could have pulled and tugged on that thread, and eventually something would have given. I was sure there was no needle attached to this thread—the X-rays would have shown that, and I'd looked twice. And there were no abutments inside the cat between her stomach—where I was now—and her mouth.

Still, gentle tension met with strong resistance. I needed to approach this from another angle.

"Becky, would you get one of those small feeding tubes and pass it into the stomach from your end?"

After some discussion over whether it would reach, we finally settled on a length of narrow plastic tubing. She used a scalpel blade to puncture a hole through one end, then slipped it over the sleeping cat's tongue until the end emerged from my incision. I tied the end of the thread through the plastic and she pulled it back.

By now most of the veterinarians reading this have figured out exactly what had happened. But I had looked into that cat's mouth—twice—and it never occurred to me. I'd even checked under the tongue, as a matter of course. I hadn't expected to find anything, and I didn't. Even though it was there.

Somehow poor Snowball had swallowed nearly three feet of sewing thread, and in the process gotten a loop caught around the base of her tongue. Over the several days preceding her hospitalization, as her body did its best to pass the unwelcome material through, the filament had cut like fine wire into the soft

tissue and vanished. A careful inspection would undoubtedly have revealed a fissure where it lay, leading to an early diagnosis.

Was I remiss? Perhaps. In my defense, I will state that on at least two occasions, while sitting in darkened halls listening to veterinary specialists discuss surgical techniques, I have seen slides of linear foreign bodies caught under cats' tongues that lie unsuspected until the time of surgery. The moral of the story is "always look under the tongue." One such lecture had taken place only months before I saw Snowball. I looked. She fought. I didn't see.

Which may have been the best thing that ever happened to her. Tugging on the thread would never have dislodged it—surgery was still the only way that was ever coming out. Had I seen it that first night, I would have had an immediate diagnosis and been able to tell the Lopez family their cat needed surgery. She would first have required rehydration and stabilization, and a total of several days in the hospital. Little would have been done differently. The bill would have approached a thousand dollars, maybe more. Snowball would have been euthanized.

Instead, I treated a cat with vague symptoms and followed the same course of diagnostics and eventual surgery she would have needed anyway. I was angry with myself when I realized what had happened, but my oversight saved Snowball's life.

Mr. Lopez was again quietly thankful when I called to explain what we found. He wasn't sure where the sewing thread had come from, but with two small boys in the house it's not hard to imagine some possibilities. We made arrangements for them to pick their cat up the following night.

They arrived once again dressed to go out, the boys clean and well-behaved. "We'll need to make arrangements," he said. And for the first time, "How much did this come to?"

"I told you I would only charge you a hundred dollars," I said, "And that's how much it is. I consider it a learning case."

With quiet dignity he paid the bill, in cash. Snowball greeted the boys with the same subdued enthusiasm I associated with the entire family. The boys were beaming as they struggled to carry her box to the car.

* * *

Ten days later, exactly on schedule, the whole family arrived once again. It was time to remove Snowball's stitches. This time she fought when I removed her from her carrier. She growled when Sharon held her on her back and I snipped the sutures from her fully healed incision. She had already put on weight, and her hair was growing back in a fuzzy down.

Smiling, I watched her leap irritably for the safety of her crate. Mr. Lopez turned to his younger son, who held a wicker basket filled with green plants. "Benny?" he prompted.

The boy blushed. He could not look at me as he held up the basket. "These are for you," he said.

"Thank you for saving our cat," said the older boy, whose name I never learned.

Fighting a grin, I matched their solemn expressions. "You're very welcome," I said.

Mr. Lopez was smiling fondly at his sons. He had graduated to canes, but the kids lugged the cat between them. They carried their burden proudly.

A Hero
Named Kiwi

Every now and then I had a chance to do a good thing, while doing very little.

One quiet Sunday night—Superbowl Sunday, actually—we received a call from the Palm Springs Police Department. This was not unusual—the police frequently brought us sick or injured strays, and I heard they vied for these short assignments, since our clinic was located near an In-N-Out Hamburgers, and the officers liked to stop there on their way back to Palm Springs. However, this call was different.

"Police dog, shot while helping to apprehend a suspect," was all the dispatcher told us. We did not know how badly the dog was injured. We prepared for the worst: IV catheter ready, blood warming for transfusion, oxygen, anesthesia machine handy in case emergency surgery was needed.

The dog walked in. He was muzzled and clearly charged with adrenaline. And he was covered with blood. At first glance it was not easy to tell where the blood was coming from.

The officer escorting the dog was not his handler. This seemed like a bad sign at first, but the officer filled us in as much as he could. The rest of the story became public knowledge within hours.

Apparently some people take the Superbowl a little too seriously. In this case, a man became incensed when his neighbor's friends parked in front of his house in order to attend a Superbowl party at the neighbor's house. The man was upset to the point he got out a gun and waved it at the offending parkers. The neighbor called police.

Now, Palm Springs is a fairly quiet town. Complaints to the local emergency line of "person has a gun" are not infrequent, but cops have learned that these complaints are usually over-reactions. The "gun" often turns out to be a toy or some totally unrelated object. But police are always alert when responding to such calls. There is always a chance the caller knows what he's talking about. Such was the case in this instance.

Three cars, one officer per car, responded to the call. One was the Canine Unit. It's a small town; they arrived within minutes of the call.

Sure enough, on the manicured lawn of his expensive home, a man stood brandishing a handgun. He waved it in the direction of his neighbor's house, shouting obscenities and demanding that the cars be moved.

The officers drew their weapons and ordered the man to drop his. The man turned his gun on the police.

The dog, Kiwi, was sent to disarm the man. The man shot Kiwi. The dog, in pain but not stopped, got up again and went after him.

By that time the man was dead.

It's hard to explain the bond between an officer and his canine partner. I'm sure I don't understand it myself. But hearing the shot, seeing the dog fall, all three men opened fire on the man. It was by-the-book police procedure. They shot to kill.

I do not know if the man was influenced by drugs, or was mentally ill, or if his behavior was caused by other personal problems. I'm sure that came out later. He was a retired physician and all reports are that nothing in his history was consistent with such an incident.

At any rate, the officers on the scene could not leave to take Kiwi to the clinic. Another car was dispatched to do that. So when I saw the dog I did not have much of the story. I only knew Kiwi had been sent after a suspect, the suspect had shot him, and been shot in return.

It wasn't easy to get an IV started because the dog, deprived of his master after hearing gunfire and being wounded himself, was less than cooperative. He did not have the emotional response of a human, that *"Oh, my God, I've been shot!"* that sends a person into shock out of proportion to the degree of injury in many cases. He did not try to bite; he just didn't want to hold still. The officer who had brought him in assisted, and we finally got the catheter in.

By now the dog was settling down, perhaps weakening as a result of lost blood. I was able to identify the entrance wound, a tiny hole at the base of Kiwi's neck. Thinking the bullet must have entered his chest cavity and that we'd be dealing with a collapsed lung at a minimum, I shaved the wound and cleaned it with antiseptic. Then we x-rayed his chest.

No bullet. A few small fragments near the entry site, but that was it. Also, the lungs looked fine. There was no blood, and no air leakage into the pleural space.

"That's weird," I said. There was so much blood I had not found the exit wound. By now I had blood all over my arms and clothes, and it had not yet occurred to me it might not have originated from the dog. The blood was mostly on Kiwi's front end, and I'd found no bloody gaping hole anywhere else.

"Okay, he was leaping or at least running at the time he was shot, right?" The officer said he was. I inserted a gloved finger slightly into the entrance wound, extending Kiwi's foreleg. The dog did not protest. This gave me an idea of the bullet's trajectory. My finger was pointing beneath the scapula, along the rib cage and toward the back of the animal's shoulder.

The exit wound was not much larger than the entrance wound. It was hidden by hair, and was not nearly as bloody as the entrance wound. The bullet had dissected between muscle layers, missed any number of major blood vessels and nerves, not fractured any bones, and passed harmlessly out through the skin.

I placed a couple of skin staples in each wound, started the dog on antibiotics and kept him overnight on IV fluids. He did fine.

The next morning the story appeared in *The Desert Sun*. For several days, the clinic received calls from members of the public asking where the dog was. They were concerned about his recovery, and often said, "My dog wants to send him a get-well card." They were told that Kiwi was recovering at home.

Over a year later, in the process of writing my first mystery novel, I called PSPD and requested a ride-along with Kiwi's handler, Don Craiger. I didn't realize at the time it was a special privilege, that Canine Units generally don't allow ride-alongs because it confuses the dog. But Kiwi was an old pro by now, and Officer Craiger figured he could handle it.

You'd never know anything had happened. He clearly enjoyed

his work, spent the whole eight-hour shift eagerly looking for action. And Officer Craiger told me something I had not realized before.

Kiwi was the first canine officer in the state to be shot in the line of duty and return to work. The small part I played in his recovery made me proud.

Wiggles:
Murphy's Law
Of Heatstroke

In veterinary medicine, even veterinary emergency medicine, there are very few true emergencies—I mean the heart-pounding kind, where minutes matter, the drop-everything-and-save-a-life kind. Bleeding arteries come to mind, but are thankfully rare. A few heart cases, choking dogs, occasionally a severely asthmatic cat might fall into this category. But by far the most dramatic case I can think of is full-blown heatstroke.

It should surprise no one that this condition is common in the Coachella Valley, where summer temperatures routinely exceed 120 degrees Fahrenheit. What is surprising—at first—is which breeds are most often affected. Given the number of long-haired dogs, such as German shepherds, cocker spaniels, and especially chow chows—*black* chow chows—who live here, I'm constantly amazed at how few of them succumb. That thick coat is as effective at insulating the dog from heat as it is from the cold.

One Sunday, Animal Control brought me two dogs they had removed from a parked car in a restaurant parking lot, probably only twenty minutes after the owners went inside. They were from out of town, as is usually the case for animals locked in cars. People passing through simply don't realize that temperatures inside these vehicles rapidly reach 150 degrees or more. And that can be fatal fast.

In this particular case, one dog was a long-haired but laid-back shepherd and the other a typical, hyperactive dalmatian. The dalmatian was dead before they got him out of the car, his skin and internal organs already blotchy from hemorrhage. The shepherd's temperature at the scene was 110, according to Animal Control officer Esther Petersen, but the restaurant had a pond and the dog was placed in shallow water and cooled off rapidly. By the time I saw him he was basically normal. Same car, vastly different outcomes.

These two cases illustrate opposite ends of a spectrum. Heat-stroke results in any species when the body's ability to cool itself is overwhelmed. Dogs don't sweat, they pant, which is much more efficient. However, body temperature depends on more than the temperature in the immediate environment; at least as important is the body heat that must be gotten rid of.

Several factors contribute to an animal's susceptibility to heat. Fur insulation is one. Another is excitability: Dalmatians as a group are active and become more so when upset. Calm dogs generate less internal heat. Another consideration is muzzle length: a longer snout cools the air as it passes through. The fourth variable is muscle-to-body-fat ratio. Muscle generates heat; therefore muscular, lean dogs are much more prone to heat-stroke than are their sedentary, overweight counterparts.

And the least tangible factor is common sense. Some dogs know when to stop and rest, get a drink of water, wade in it if possible. Other dogs literally do not have the sense to come out of the sun. (It's interesting to note that I've never treated a cat for this condition!)

Recall Frannie the boxer, who staggered in through the doggy door when the owner came home from work, only to collapse onto the air-conditioned tile floor with a temperature of 112. The air had been on all day. The doggy door had been open. Clearly, the dog knew where the door was located. But she almost died because it didn't occur to her to come inside earlier.

She was a boxer. Short-haired, athletic, blunt-nosed and absolutely lacking in thought processes, boxers make up a good twenty percent of the heatstroke cases I've seen.

Don't get me wrong. I *love* boxers. How can you not love anything so enthusiastic? So happy. So completely forgiving. But their owners just don't realize the risk of heatstroke, and every year we see at least one case.

Wiggles was the worst. She had been out jogging with Tanya, the young girl who owned her. Tanya rode her bicycle. Wiggles barely made it home.

Dr. Nancy Carlson was on duty when Wiggles arrived. The

dog was comatose, gasping for breath, her gums a dramatic deep purple. Nancy immediately started an IV, pumping in the fluids we kept refrigerated for that purpose. An oxygen line provided relief for her starved tissues, then dexamethasone for shock, a powerful antibiotic, and heparin to prevent bleeding.

Actually, heparin prevents clotting, which on its surface appears to be the opposite of bleeding. But what happens in heatstroke is the tissues are literally cooking. The damage is intense, and the body's natural defense is to form clots where damage occurs, and later go back to repair things more completely. But with injury this severe, the demand on the clotting system is enormous, quickly exhausting available supplies of the chemicals known as coagulation factors. The heat further denatures these proteins, and the coagulation system collapses. Once that happens even minor trauma—of which there is plenty in these cases—leads to hemorrhage. The animal (it happens in people, too) literally bleeds to death without a wound. The technical name for this syndrome is disseminated intravascular coagulopathy, abbreviated DIC. This abbreviation has been cynically expanded to what was traditionally believed to be its more realistic definition: Death Is Coming.

DIC and brain damage, either from direct thermal injury or subsequent edema, or swelling, are the usual causes of death in heatstroke. And this one was bad. Her temperature exceeded 112 at the time of presentation. Illogically, it had probably gone up during the trip to the clinic, due to the inefficient panting and muscle stiffness that occurs. But temperatures of that magnitude for any length of time can't help but damage the brain.

As soon as she could turn away from her patient, Nancy explained the poor prognosis to Samantha, Tanya's mother. Tanya might be Wiggles's owner, but Samantha had to pay the bill. Samantha was a nurse, with intensive care experience, and understood what Nancy was saying. She understood that it would be expensive, and the bill would have to be paid even if treatment didn't work. She was not wealthy, but she was committed to Wiggles. And to her daughter. Wiggles was a replacement dog for one that had been put to sleep two years earlier after being run over by a car; her husband had left her a year later, and Samantha knew her daughter needed the stability of canine sameness.

Wiggles was a family member, and Samantha could not turn her back on the dog and still face her daughter.

So the intensive process of attempting to save Wiggles began. By now, ironically, her body temperature had plummeted into the subnormal range, which Nancy had anticipated. This is the reason we no longer soak these dogs in cold water: For twenty-four hours or so, Wiggles's body would not be able to regulate its own temperature. It's much easier to warm a dry dog than a wet one.

So she was wrapped in blankets, with heating pads over and under, and switched first to room-temperature fluids and then to plasma. Plasma is the clear portion of whole blood, collected from healthy dogs and frozen until needed. It contains lifesaving clotting factors, and is thicker than so-called crystalloid fluids, thereby helping, via osmosis, to pull edema fluid from the brain and shrink its swelling.

Wiggles gradually regained consciousness over the course of the night. She remained depressed, but by the following morning, when I came on duty, she recognized Tanya and Samantha readily, her four-inch tail stub proving her name. If she had brain damage, no one could tell.

Fortunately it was Saturday of Memorial Day weekend, so Wiggles would receive round-the-clock care for three days, without the need to move her to another facility.

Despite multiple plasma transfusions and thrice-daily administration of heparin, Wiggles developed moderate DIC. The most vulnerable organ system, but fortunately the mostly easily treated, is the intestinal tract. By Sunday afternoon Wiggles was vomiting blood and passing foul bloody diarrhea. The entire clinic reeked of it, and the staff was challenged trying to keep clean blankets available. Samantha was again offered the option of euthanasia. It was tougher for her this time, because Wiggles was clearly uncomfortable. But pain is something we can treat. Again she elected to continue. More drugs were added to the regimen, to control abdominal pain and in a futile effort to staunch the diarrhea.

Wiggles's temperature stabilized at around 103, a slight fever (normal for dogs ranges from 100 to 102). We switched antibiotics in hopes of warding off potentially fatal infections.

Samantha sat with her for hours at a time. Tanya stayed away, anticipating the worst.

By Monday morning Wiggles had stopped vomiting and the diarrhea had dropped off to one severe episode every eight hours or so. Her temperature hovered at 103, and she showed no inclination to take food or water. But the body can go a long time without food, and we were taking care of her water needs. Plasma and clear fluids sustained her.

Of new concern was evidence from the lab tests that Wiggles's kidneys were being affected. All the toxins from her damaged tissues were bombarding the kidneys and basically clogging them up. So far she was making adequate urine. All I could do was turn up the rate of her fluids in hopes of giving her overburdened kidneys enough water to flush away the poison. And a diuretic went on the treatment list.

Samantha continued to visit, twice a day, sitting cross-legged in the run with Wiggles's head in her lap until her knees and back ached. Often one or both of the resident cats curled up with them. Red and Tex frequently lay next to sick animals; some appeared to take comfort from them.

Tuesday morning we faced a dilemma. The emergency clinic closed from eight to five. We could leave Wiggles unattended, still connected to the pump that regulated her fluid rate. Her medications could easily be arranged around the hours we were gone. Or we could transfer her to a daytime clinic.

This is a quandary I faced often during my tenure. I had learned that most veterinarians, and most clinics, simply weren't equipped to handle cases like Wiggles. Even the best local practices at the time lacked IV pumps, plasma, in-house laboratory equipment, and the ability to monitor a critical patient well. Most are set up for reasonably healthy pets. But now Wiggles was receiving constant IV fluids, daily plasma transfusion, daily lab work—some parameters were being checked three times a day—heparin, antibiotics, painkillers, a diuretic, anti-inflammatories and an H2 blocker, Zantac. Some needed to be given twice a day, others three times. It was a delicate balance. Their effects had to be monitored. Her urine output bore watching. The staffs at most clinics are too busy to deal with so needy a patient, and subtle changes in condition can easily be missed. This does not speak badly of my colleagues or their staffs; it's simply a divergence of focus.

Unfortunately, many of the vets in question genuinely don't realize what the profession is capable of. Egos get in the way, as do economics. I was under strict orders to transfer every case to another vet, every morning, except by specific arrangement with that vet. Most were never sent back, but remained at the other clinic, left alone overnight. I also felt it was in Wiggles's best interest not to change vets just then, because her case was so complex and I was most familiar with it.

I discussed the options at length with Samantha. She could take Wiggles to her regular vet and insist she return to us overnight. Or she could leave Wiggles alone at our clinic until we reopened at five o'clock. But by now the dog, though still obviously sick, was looking like a survivor. And, frankly, the bill was mounting. Samantha decided to leave Wiggles at the emergency clinic until evening.

The issue was made simpler by the fact that Samantha felt no particular allegiance to the vet who had given Wiggles her annual vaccinations. She decided Nancy would be her new doctor, so the arrangements were easy. I got Nancy's enthusiastic permission to keep her, left Wiggles hooked up to her pump and went home for a much-needed nap.

That evening I returned half-fearing the worst. I hurried into the treatment area holding my breath. Wiggles looked up tiredly from her clean blanket, and when she saw me immediately struggled to her feet and proved that she still had intestinal problems, and her bladder was working just fine. She had refused to soil her bedding until someone was available to clean up after her. I had to laugh.

She was still tired, and spent most of her time sleeping. But she took some water, and responded eagerly to affection. The lab work showed that her kidneys were holding their own, and her electrolytes were stable. Her clotting time was still prolonged, but no worse than the previous evening.

That night even Tanya visited. Wiggles showed more animation when she saw her best friend than she had all weekend. I began to allow myself to think she would eventually go home.

Wiggles remained at the emergency clinic until Friday morning. Each day her attitude improved slightly. Each night as Samantha sat with her, Wiggles passed bloody diarrhea like foul floodwaters, but her lab work said she was healing. Even her kidneys had stabilized. Every night she got her plasma, and on Wednesday night, when her packed cell volume dropped too low from the constant blood loss, she received one unit of whole blood. She was the first heatstroke I'd ever had to transfuse with cells, but it made all the difference. Thursday morning she ate for the first time. For twenty-four hours she passed no feces at all, then they came out nearly normal.

For two days before she went home, Wiggles developed a swelling in the leg that held her IV line. This IV line had replaced the original, which had clotted on Tuesday, and there was no easy place for a new one, so we left it where it was.

On Friday morning when I pulled it and sent her home on oral antibiotics, I was convinced the swelling would disappear now that the leg was not bandaged. However, when I saw her the following Sunday—over a week after the original episode—she was still subdued, still not eating well. Her temperature was back up, at 103 again. And there was pus draining from the old IV site.

The leg had developed phlebitis, an infection of a vein. Her white blood cell count (WBC) was high, confirming the presence of infection, but the anemia had apparently gone for good. She was no longer losing blood through her intestines, and her bone marrow was in good shape to crank out new cells. There was nothing to do but continue the antibiotics, feed protein-rich food to encourage healing, and apply warm compresses to the leg several times daily. Either the leg would heal, or the infection would overwhelm her defenses and send us on another rescue mission.

The following Tuesday night I rechecked her again. She was much brighter, the swelling had gone down, the drainage cleared up, and her temperature was normal. Likewise her kidney function remained normal. Her appetite had improved and her WBC had come down, though it was still above normal. She had gained weight, though she still appeared skeletal. I sent her home to return in three days.

That was Friday night. One week after Wiggles had been re-leased from the clinic, almost two weeks following the original heatstroke, all our efforts were rewarded. In through the door walked a normal young boxer. A boxer who lived up to her name. A boxer with a scar on her leg, where the hair was just beginning to grow back. With normal lab results and a normal temperature. A boxer with a tremendous appetite and lots of weight to gain back after her ordeal.

I never saw Wiggles again after that. Tanya would be a young adult now, Wiggles middle-aged. I hope the dog still sleeps at the foot of her mistress's bed.

And I hope she stays indoors in summer.

Not So Different
From Me

I had been working at the emergency clinic for about three and a half years before I attended a conference devoted to the subject.

I've always loved veterinary conventions. I make a point of attending at least one major meeting a year, and one or two smaller ones—the latter generally devoted to a single subject such as heart disease or gastroenterology. I'd been to the California Veterinary Medical Association annual meeting the year before, and to the annual conference of The American College of Veterinary Surgeons two years ago. I never failed to come home with renewed enthusiasm for my profession. New techniques, new drugs, new equipment are introduced at such gatherings. Impromptu discussions with colleagues in the exhibit hall or over snacks between lectures often yield practice tips that make established tasks easier.

But so far nothing had led me to consider emergency practice a career. I'd been practicing it for three years, but only in the broadest sense. In school I'd been taught a systematic diagnostic-and-treatment protocol, and my internship reinforced that. The emergency clinic certainly attracted a high percentage of very sick animals, without the wellness exams and vaccination visits to break things up. But I had given little thought to this fact. I just went to work every night and tried to do my best, with the support of almost thirty referring veterinarians, each of whom had his or her own ideas of what we should be doing.

The emergency clinician holds a unique position within the veterinary community. Many, if not most, of our clients would prefer to be seeing their regular DVM. The practice I worked in was owned by a corporation formed by those same veterinarians. Their primary goal in establishing AEC was to enable them to take nights and weekends off without worrying about patient emergencies. It required an enormous degree of cooperation between professionals who could rarely agree on anything specific. There is a truism: Ask three vets how to do something, and you'll get four opinions.

Some assumed we would always remain basically a first aid station, doing the minimum to keep our patients going until the referring vets opened the next day—thus delivering animals back to them prepared for surgery or diagnostic testing or whatever was indicated. Others envisioned it as a pressure valve—a place to send emergency surgical cases or high-maintenance medical ones they were too busy to deal with. Most took their turns on duty when it first opened. The different expectations were never addressed.

But with the new affordability of first-rate equipment, a strange metamorphosis was taking place. During the course of two years or so we were transformed from a minimally staffed clinic with hodgepodge materials into the best-equipped facility in the valley. It took courage and faith for those veterinarians to allow this co-owned hospital, staffed by their employees, to eclipse them both in diagnostic and case-management capability. It made perfect sense to do so—we had a much higher percentage of severely ill pets who could not wait for test results. We were centrally located and available for referral if they wanted to take advantage of what they had bought us. Lives were unquestionably saved as a result of these machines. And that would seem, on the surface, to be everyone's ultimate goal.

But practice owners must also be businesspeople. They are human beings with egos and insecurities. We were asking them to trust us, not only with the animals they cared for but with the clients who were their livelihood.

Every referral reflected on the referring vet. Their judgment was evaluated, however fairly, by each client based on the quality of care we were perceived to provide. In this way the improvements benefited everyone.

However, the clients were also comparing services. They came to us during times of high stress, often unable to remember their own vets' names. We took over and managed whatever crisis they brought. The bond they felt with us was sometimes stronger than the one with the person who gave Fluffy her annual shots and might have cleaned her teeth a couple of times.

Also, each blood panel, every radiograph, IV catheter, and operation we performed was one that would not be done by someone else. This translates in a real and immediately tangible way into loss of income for this other vet. Some handled it better than others.

I was employed by these people; I had to answer to all of them. But I also needed to keep the clients happy, and their concerns were much more immediate. The referring vets didn't always agree with me on how a case should be managed. I became reluctant to refer back to them in certain instances. Sometimes the stress of pleasing my colleagues overshadowed the stress of treating the patients.

Every other October the International Veterinary Emergency and Critical Care Symposium takes place in San Antonio, Texas. The first was in 1988—this was not an old discipline. The very idea of high-tech veterinary medicine was somewhat new, and the profession was far from united behind the concept. Some saw these facilities as a threat; others welcomed their specialization.

For me, attending IVECCS III meant a commitment to both my job and the expanding discipline of emergency medicine.

It was a revelation.

I had begun to feel our little emergency clinic was pretty well-equipped. By local standards, that was true. I even entertained the notion that I was getting good at my job. And our survival rate was undeniably rising. But all the things I didn't know! Never suspected were possible! I spent every hour in lecture halls, discovering the wonders of colloid therapy, new heart medication borrowed from human medicine, ventilation, central venous pressure monitoring, gastrostomy tube management.

Between lectures I met people like myself—young, for the most part, full of enthusiasm for their work. People for whom blood gas measurements and serum osmolality did not cause the eyes to glaze. Practitioners on the cutting edge.

So much had changed since I graduated—only five years earlier! But, oddly, for the first time in my life I felt as if I belonged. The excitement my colleagues felt extended to me—we were all lucky to be part of veterinary medicine at that moment. Better yet, we were part of an elite group for whom the worst cases, the ones our saner colleagues dreaded most, spelled an opportunity to try new things. After all, if it looked like a lost cause, nothing we could do would hurt—so any reasonable treatment was worth a try. Here, then, were others like me, who recalled not the ones that got away but the ones that lived, the ones that went home against all odds. And, day by day, we would change those odds.

Emergency and Critical Care was a new specialty discipline, still undergoing review by the American Veterinary Medical Association for inclusion in its list of colleges. Specialization meant official recognition—it also meant a lot of hard work.

Few residencies were available; it was still possible to become board-eligible without completing such a program. Conditions were rather vague. Thus far credentials had been offered only to pioneers in the field who were already boarded in other disciplines. A grueling exam would be offered only for those who had first met certain criteria: five years in practice; teaching within the discipline; publishing in a peer-reviewed journal or preparing detailed case reports; the best equipment; an undetermined number of hours at a critical care center—veterinary or human. M&M rounds—Morbidity and Mortality—at a teaching hospital was suggested for those who lacked access to veterinary critical care centers.

Board certification didn't necessarily mean more money. But it symbolized a higher standard, a huge accomplishment.

I thought about it. I talked to people who had done it. It would be a long road, and the details were cloudy at this point. But in the meantime, I could get my feet wet. Even if I never earned the right to affix the letters "dipl, ACVECC"—diplomate of the American College of Veterinary Emergency and Critical Care—after my "DVM," whatever knowledge I picked up in the interim could only be a good thing.

We don't have a teaching hospital in the desert. I called each of our three full-service human hospitals asking about Grand Rounds, anything that might qualify. Desert Hospital held thrice-weekly Trauma rounds. I called Trauma, and eventually spoke to a registered nurse named Anita Ciatola.

"You're a vet?" she asked, baffled but enjoying herself.

"Yep. I'm thinking of going for specialization in emergency and critical care, and part of the requirement is to attend rounds at a critical care facility."

We talked about the details a little bit and she said, "We start at nine. Come in a little early Monday and I'll show you around."

Anita's official title was Director of Trauma Services. She ran the place. We became friends until nearly three years later, when she moved to Arizona and we lost touch.

For the next two years—seasons, actually, since they were suspended for the summer—I attended Trauma Rounds. We met at approximately nine A.M. in Trauma Critical Care. Any given session might be attended by the nurses on duty, student nurses, pharmacology students, nutritionists, almost anyone involved in patient care. Dr. Frank Ercoli, one of the trauma surgeons, made me feel welcome. He had instigated the rounds sessions in an effort to stimulate a learning environment. I think he regretted not having residents.

The CCU—Critical Care Unit—was a roughly octagonal room, a door in each wall leading to a patient room. We moved from room to room, discussing the patient's condition and any complications that might have arisen since the previous session. Dr. Ercoli, as tall and arrogant as any surgeon, also had a keen sense of humor and a well-honed radar for those who were not paying attention.

"How will you know when this patient has a pulmonary thromboembolism?" he might ask the nurse assigned to the patient in question.

It wasn't meanness. The nurse, unable to answer, might resent the spotlight. But the next time he or she would be prepared.

I learned about silent aspiration and pneumonia, pulmonary thromboembolism, renal infarct. I drooled over the ease with which CT scans were obtained, and learned their value in assessing internal injuries. I marveled over the worth of human life, the extremes to which modern medicine could go to preserve it—and the agony involved in failure. I listened to discussions about the cost of albumen vs. Hetastarch, alcohol drips to prevent addicted patients from going through withdrawal while their bodies dealt with life-threatening trauma. I absorbed the sobering statistics on impaired drivers and automobile accidents.

Small details of certain cases come back to me: the tourist who had posed for a picture beside a palm tree, only to have the tree suddenly topple over. It would have been funny had it not broken several bones, including three in her spine. There was a man who had led police on a high-speed chase, which ended when he collided with an elderly woman. Both entered T-CCU that night. The woman lived; the man eventually did not. During the two weeks he was there I listened to debates on how far they should go to save him. For them this was only a medical issue; for me the morality was impossible to escape. I felt for the first time how hard it is to separate the person from the patient.

I watched a colostomy operation on a woman who had been shot with a shotgun by her boyfriend; observed the intake procedure as a dozen or more masked and gowned figures descended on a naked man brought in by paramedics after falling from a roof. (He wasn't naked when he fell—the paramedics had cut away his clothing.) I felt his fear as fingers and instruments and catheters and needles penetrated every orifice and created new ones.

I sat in on a vote—whether a comatose, jaundiced man with a severely infected incision following abdominal surgery should be resuscitated when he coded. Not "if" he coded. When. Fortunately, the only votes that really counted were those of the surgeons in charge and the man's family.

In the long run, I decided not to pursue board certification. Specialization would mean recognition, and a major sense of accomplishment. But it is also limiting to some extent—a permanent bond to emergency work—and I was beginning to chafe at being an employee. However, I will never regret any of the time I spent following Dr. Ercoli's long strides down the corridors of Desert Hospital.

Many of my colleagues seem to resent our MD counterparts. They bristle when asked, "Why didn't you become a *real* doctor?" The answer, of course, is that we *are* real doctors—our patients just happen to be animals.

I have heard of quite a few veterinarians who, frustrated with the constraints placed on them by clients who could not pay for their skills, went on to medical school. Over the years, I have had three medical doctors tell me that, if they were starting today, they would choose veterinary medicine over human medicine. I am grateful to have chosen the correct path for myself.

My maternal grandfather, whom I never met because he died before I was born, was a physician. My stepfather is a pediatrician—we tell some of the same stories. I now have numerous clients who are doctors of varying types. Some are delightful clients, others are insufferable. In short, they are all human.

And not so different from me.

That Dog Don't Hunt

"Do whatever you can, Doc." We both studied the bleeding face of his unconscious pointer. "My wife is going to kill me."

Specks was bred for hunting, and that's exactly what he'd been doing when he was shot. But the eight-year-old German short-haired pointer spent most of his time as a house pet, and on this year's annual Saturday dove-hunting expedition he had forgotten the hunting dog's cardinal rule: You're only supposed to *flush* the birds, you do *not* leap up after them.

Unfortunately Jeff Burrows didn't hunt any more than his dog did, and lacked the reflexes to avoid the shot. By the time he realized the dog was in the way, he'd already pulled the trigger. A load of birdshot caught the dog square in the head. Specks dropped like a stone.

He was still unconscious when they got to the clinic, at least forty-five minutes after the accident. A deep furrow carved its way down Specks's face, taking out much of his forehead but leaving the bone underneath apparently undamaged. Judging from the size and angle of the groove, I guessed the shot had been close-range but glancing. It had taken skin and muscle and fascia from the forehead but left his muzzle relatively undamaged.

"His odds aren't good," I said. "Even if he survives, he'll probably be blind." The cornea of the left eye had been perforated, and the whole eye would eventually need to be removed. I could not predict the degree of brain damage the dog might have suffered besides.

Mr. Burrows said he understood. "Do everything you can," he said. "He doesn't have to be able to hunt, he's a good old dog. My wife. . . . Do whatever you can."

182

I had already initiated treatment for pain and brain edema and infection—the ubiquitous fluids and steroids and antibiotics, since this was long before I'd ever heard of Hetastarch. So I wrote up a quick estimate, turned him over to the front desk, and asked him to wait while I took X-rays.

Dogs have pretty small brains relative to the size of their heads. The bone itself is thick and laced with an extensive network of sinuses, so it takes a lot of trauma to actually breach the skull. I figured some of the buckshot had lodged in the frontal sinuses, but the films showed an undamaged layer of cortex. Only a few pieces of shot dotted the heavy muscle that remained above the ears. The concussion Specks was clearly suffering from resulted from the impact of fast-moving pellets, and possibly a *contre-coup* injury as he fell, rather than direct trauma.

This was good news. In fact, the dog was already beginning to stir.

Before he fully regained consciousness, I infiltrated the wound with local anesthetic and sutured it closed as best I could. A fair amount of tissue was missing, but I was able to close most of the gap. I applied an antiseptic ointment to the rest to protect it from the air so it wouldn't hurt so much. Becky actually had to hold him still by the time I finished.

Mr. Burrows was ecstatic. Or as nearly so as possible given the circumstances. The dog wasn't yet responding to his name, but was clearly regaining awareness of his surroundings. I hoped privately the blast hadn't also damaged the animal's ears.

Mr. Burrows declined my offer of the phone to call his wife and explain. "Is there a florist nearby?" he asked. The staff was able to direct him to the nearest one. He was anxious but relieved when he left.

Specks continued to improve overnight. First he rolled onto his chest, clearly confused by the strange odors and the tile floor beneath his blanket and the IV in his leg. With great relief I saw him twitch his ears and move his head in the direction of my voice when I called his name. He started to get up, so I moved over to his run to try to soothe him. I ran my hand down his neck, his back, under his chin, careful to avoid his face. His muscular body quivered. His last memory was of leaping after dove. To him it must have felt like being suddenly transported from a normal, joyous activity—pointer heaven—to a dark and terrifying hell. With a splitting headache (so to speak).

It is said, and is probably true, that sight is the least important of the senses as far as dogs are concerned. Certainly his breed depends more on smell and hearing. But dogs, like other species, rely on vision to steer them around objects, over defects in their path, after distant rabbits. I'd known blind dogs before, and some did better than others. Specks would not have the benefit of cataracts that developed slowly while he learned to avoid running into furniture that grew increasingly indistinct. His blindness was immediate and complete. And he had awakened in a strange place, surrounded by people he'd never met before. And unlike a human in the same situation, he could not understand our explanations.

But he didn't complain. From the beginning, even before it became clear that Specks's brain was as functional as it had ever been, he seemed to understand his new limitations and accept them. Blindness was inconvenient, especially for a dog of his class. But he couldn't do anything about that, so he set out to learn how to be a blind dog.

By the time the Burrowses visited late Sunday morning, Specks was going for leash walks, maneuvering the turns and doorways with only occasional collisions. It's possible his lacerated and painful face gave him incentive not to bump into things—that *hurt!* But he was clearly an exceptionally intelligent animal.

Being reunited with his owners made a big difference. Whatever residual depression I'd seen evaporated when he realized he was not abandoned to the vet. His posture changed—his tense, head-down stance relaxed and the head came up, the two-inch tail stub waving joyfully as if to say, "All is forgiven. I know you didn't mean it."

In fact, by that afternoon, I had no reason to keep him any longer. I released him to his owners. It was fascinating to watch him stop at the tailgate of the pickup he'd ridden in so many times, calculate the distance, and place his front feet up in the bed. Mr. Burrows lifted him from there, and climbed in to ride home with him while his wife drove. It was a good arrangement, but I had the feeling Specks would soon be jumping in without help.

Jala Peño

"Is my bird supposed to be lying on the bottom of his cage?"

It wasn't the first time I'd heard this question over the phone. The answer is pretty obvious, though. "Are you sure he's still breathing? Then get him in here now!"

These birds sometimes arrive dead. If they are still alive, the prognosis is very poor—they are simply too far gone to survive. Birds in the wild are prey animals; in other words, they are food for other, larger animals. For this reason they will instinctively "pretend" to be healthy for as long as possible. Unwary bird owners often don't realize their pets are sick until it is too late to help them.

Jala was almost dead, and as Mr. Peño had only owned him a few days, I assumed it would be a euthanasia. But I was wrong. "Please try to help him," he insisted. He said he understood what I was saying, that it was all but hopeless. "Please do everything you can."

I asked how long Jala had been sick. He said the bird had not been sick at all, until he found him unconscious. Jala's physical examination, not surprisingly, proved this wrong. His keel, or breast bone, jutted sharply. The bird was emaciated.

Part of the history was gone forever, as Jala—a red-lored Amazon parrot whose head had been dyed a spectacular blue—had been purchased from a street vendor in Mexico and smuggled back to California the week before. Tourists spot the hapless birds in tiny wire cages and feel sorry for them. Importing parrots is, of course, illegal when done in this manner, but not difficult. Mr. Peño had received Jala as a gift, and had taken the bird to an avian vet the next day. I knew I'd be able to reach the vet the next morning. In the meantime, I had a lot of work to do.

I carried the moribund bird to the back room and placed him in an incubator, with oxygen flowing in, while I got what I needed. First I gave him what I think of as my "sick bird cocktail"— something for everyone when you don't have time to wait for diagnostic tests. It contained some B vitamins, some calcium, the tiniest bit of short-acting dexamethasone for shock, an antibiotic, and fluids. I gave it intravenously, and included a little glucose for good measure.

But intravenous injections are problematic in birds because their fragile veins won't tolerate indwelling catheters, and repeated injections require handling that can stress a sick patient past the point of tolerance—in other words, the treatment can kill it. And it was clear this bird would require more injections as the night progressed.

The solution was obvious. Jala would need an intra-osseous canula—a catheter placed into a bone in his wing, a technique introduced not so long ago in very young puppies and kittens, or any animal whose veins were too small and fragile to take a catheter. I'd put them in kittens and puppies. I'd once put one into the femur of a baby potbellied pig. I'd sat through lectures and glanced through articles that demonstrated how to use them in parrots. I had never been called upon to use that knowledge. But it was Jala's only chance.

The fact that my patient was comatose helped. With the latest avian text lying open on the treatment table and looking at the pictures as much as at Jala, I laid him on a towel, plucked a few feathers and prepared the area with antiseptic. Using a 22-gauge needle I attempted to slip it into Jala's bone. It stuck on cortex. I pushed harder. The needle bounced off bone, slid through unresisting wing tissue and hard into my thumb. I muttered something unprofessional and turned my attention toward stemming the blood flow in my hand. I'd rammed the needle to my own bone, and it wouldn't do to bleed all over my patient.

Since I'm terribly allergic to adhesives, I wrapped a crude bandage of gauze and nonstick Vetrap around my thumb and got a new needle from the drawer. The bulky bandage made handling Jala's wing awkward, but it protected my thumb from another similar episode. And I thought I knew what I'd done wrong.

Gently clasping the bone in my hand, I tried again—more slowly this time, with a twisting motion. The needle bit soft bird bone. Under pressure, it penetrated cortex. It slipped through and into the hollow medulla. The feeling is indescribable—you just know when it's right.

So far Jala hadn't moved or protested. A couple of times I'd had to check to make sure he was still breathing. I wrapped tape around the hub of the needle and sutured it to skin. I secured a short length of flexible tubing to the catheter. I drew up another syringe, this time containing mostly glucose solution, and slowly injected it through the tubing and into Jala's bone marrow cavity.

The effect was amazing. By the time I had him connected to an IV pump that would deliver more fluids continuously throughout the night, Jala was standing up. He was weak, head down and eyelids at half-mast, but was showing by far the most animation I'd seen. Clearly hypoglycemia, or low blood sugar, partially explained his condition. I wondered how long it had been since Jala had eaten. I hoped the condition was not due to liver disease or some other metabolic abnormality. I sincerely hoped the bird had succumbed to a bacterial infection and the stress of being captured, dyed, caged, and transported across the border. If he had a virus or a fungal infection, or severe liver disease, no amount of glucose and antibiotics would save him.

After placing a bandage to keep the tubing in place, I called his owner back to see. He reacted ecstatically, and I saw my mistake. Once he saw the improvement, he assumed his bird would be fine. I had to emphasize that so far I had only treated symptoms. Jala had a long way to go before he was out of the woods.

Mr. Peño said he understood, but he left with an awfully big grin on his face.

My heart felt heavy. The adrenaline rush had faded. The last thing I did was feed the Amazon, a gruel mix placed directly into his crop (a pouch in the throat where birds store food for later digestion) with a syringe and rubber tubing. Calories were crucial, and I would tube-feed him again the next morning. There was nothing much left for me to do—further handling would be detrimental. From here on out it was up to Jala.

And Jala was not an ideal patient. He was terrified. He had only been captive for a short time, and from his point of view it had been a horrible experience. He naturally assumed we planned to kill and eat him any minute. It was hands-off time. All I could do was cover most of the incubator so he couldn't see us (since he would otherwise expend energy he couldn't afford, trying to fool us into thinking he was fine) and resist the temptation to check on him frequently. Bowls of seed and Rocky's pellets and fresh fruit, donated from Becky's dinner, and water were available to him. He had fluids and oxygen and a nice warm, dark place to rest. I hoped he would feel safe enough to get better.

I left a message for Dr. Bart Huber, the avian vet in Los Angeles who had seen Jala a few days before, and tried to get some sleep. My thumb hurt and I worried that there was something I'd neglected to do, some crucial factor I'd forgotten to address. I was up early.

Jala was much stronger. Dr. Huber called and mentioned his concern about a klebsiella infection—a nasty but treatable bacteria. The antibiotic I had selected should cover that. When Mr. Peño arrived, he was thrilled to see Jala eyeing us both suspiciously. I filled his crop again, since he didn't seem to have eaten anything, gently disconnected the IV and transferred the bird to his carrying cage. He would spend the day with Dr. Doug Kunz, who would run some basic diagnostic tests to rule out more serious disease.

Cultures eventually confirmed the klebsiella infection. Jala returned that night and stayed in a regular cage. He was eating on his own—only seed at first, and a peanut grudgingly contributed by Rocky, my own African gray parrot. The following morning he went home. Mr. Peño learned how to inject the antibiotic into Jala's muscle—what little muscle he had.

Several months later a note arrived, thanking me for helping Jala pull through. Along with the note was a photograph. It showed a very-much-alive Jala, perched on a playground constructed of wooden dowels with colorful bird toys strewn everywhere. The blue had faded from his head, and his posture and expression seemed to indicate curiosity rather than fear. It looked as if Jala was adapting to his new home. I hope he lives a long and happy life.

Sometimes
You Need Help

About a year after I moved to the desert, I heard about Dan Westfall and his chimps. Dan had performing primates, including the original Cheeta from the old Johnny Weissmuller Tarzan movies, and he had recently moved to Palm Springs. I thought that was pretty interesting, and wondered briefly who he used for a veterinarian. Then I didn't think about it anymore.

A year later I bought a house in Palm Springs and moved down from Morongo Valley. I'd been renting five acres in Morongo, and I missed the openness. However, the commute had gotten old, and I'd managed to buy a fixer-upper with a large fenced yard for the dogs. I spent most of my spare time working on the house, speaking to a few of my neighbors but not really getting to know anyone. Many were renters, and turnover was high. They worked days and I worked nights, so I wasn't on more than a nodding acquaintance with anyone.

However, one neighbor caught my attention. I was heading for work one day when I passed a man on a motorcycle with what looked like two chimpanzees. I almost stopped, but I was running late and didn't have time. But I took note of where he lived—less than two blocks from me on the same street.

Over the next couple of years, I would occasionally wave as I passed. He waved back and that was it. Until one Thursday night when Becky asked me to take a phone call.

"Hello?" I said. "This is Dr. Roberts."

He sounded nervous. "I've got a little chimp who's sick," said the voice. "I know no one likes to work with them, but he isn't eating and I'm real worried."

He was right about vets not liking to work with primates. They

191

are strong and can be extremely mean. They are uncannily intelligent, and not always cooperative. And they can carry human diseases.

"He's only six. He had a cold about a week ago. I think he got it from me," the voice went on. "I'm afraid it's turned into pneumonia."

I asked a few questions and ascertained that this was the same man who lived down the street from me. I was hesitant, nervous about working with a chimp, both for the reasons listed above and because they were not familiar to me.

"I've got a vet in LA you can talk to." He gave me a name and number. I already figured I'd work on the chimp, but I told him I'd call him back.

I called the LA veterinarian for advice. The first thing he told me was, "Watch out. I know he's little and cute, but he can tear your arm off if he gets mad."

That made me pause. I'd worked with horses for a good part of my life, and horses have killed people. However, horses are relatively stupid creatures and are manageable in their way. I knew about horses, could predict their behavior in most cases. I knew nothing at all about chimps, except that they are humans' nearest relatives.

"But he's been raised by Dan his entire life! He's tame!"

"He still has chimpanzee instincts, and right now he's sick. He'll be irritable and might decide you're the reason he doesn't feel well. Don't do anything that hurts even a little bit. Listen to me. I know what I'm talking about."

"Assuming I see him, what would you recommend I do?"

"He's probably got pneumonia, like Dan says. Try Keflex."

Well, that was easy enough. But in order to prescribe medication, the law says I have to have a working relationship with the client, and have seen and examined the animal in question. I couldn't very well leave work and go to him at that point. So I called Dan back and told him to bring Jeeter to the clinic.

Jeeter was, as predicted, small and cute. Looking at him, it was hard to believe he was as strong as the vet in LA had suggested. At any rate, I hardly got close enough to find out—Dan kept himself between me and the chimp the whole time they were there—which made my job difficult, since I couldn't auscultate the chimp's lungs to confirm pneumonia. But it also made me feel safer.

"Let's x-ray his chest," I suggested. "Then I may have to send the films over to the hospital for them to read."

Getting the little chimp on the X-ray table was easy. I set everything up beforehand, and coached Dan from the doorway of the tiny room. He put on the lead apron normally worn by my staff, and lay Jeeter on his back on the table. I stepped on the foot-operated switch from just outside.

It turned out I didn't need a radiologist to tell me Jeeter did, indeed, have pneumonia. It was obvious. For another animal I would at a minimum have given an antibiotic injection to get him started, but this patient I had to treat from a distance. I prescribed the Keflex suspension, which is cherry-flavored to appeal to children, and sent Jeeter and Dan on their way with a request to let me know how he was doing the next day. And I did something I rarely do—I gave Dan my home phone number, since I was pretty sure he was right about other vets being reluctant to see Jeeter in an emergency.

But there was one small problem: Jeeter wanted nothing to do with the Keflex. He wasn't eating or drinking, and acted sicker than ever the next day. Having taken on the case, I felt obligated to do something. But what?

Okay, I told myself, pretend Jeeter's a dog. What would you do?

That was easy enough. I would hospitalize the animal and give intravenous antibiotics until the animal felt well enough to take nourishment and medication by mouth. But the drugs I normally would use need to be given three times a day, and the fluids are given continually. That wouldn't work with Jeeter.

But we had to do something, or he would continue to deteriorate and eventually die. Dan was growing distraught. "He sleeps in the bed with me," he said. "I can hear him wheezing. What are we going to do?"

The LA vet recommended anesthetizing Jeeter and treating him while he was out. The prospect terrified me. I hated the thought of putting an animal under anesthesia that was already sick, especially one having trouble breathing. Add to that my uncertainty regarding what drugs to use in the species, and I would cheerfully have sent him to Los Angeles. But the gentle voice on the phone belonged to a retired practitioner. He had no hospital. He could not see Jeeter himself.

It was dawning on me that I really had no choice. I would have to anesthetize the chimp, and the sooner the better—he was only going to get worse. And I couldn't keep him under indefinitely—we would have to plan carefully to maximize the benefits and minimize the risks.

By now of course it was Saturday. I needed advice from medical doctors, and they were scarce on weekends. Fortunately, through attending trauma rounds and work I had done with the local Institute of Critical Care Medicine, I knew a few by name. I started leaving messages. Then I called my stepfather, Richard Waldman, who is a pediatrician in North Carolina. He offered quite a lot of advice regarding intravenous rates and antibiotics I might use.

Frank Ercoli, the trauma surgeon, gave me the dosage recommendation for ketamine in children. Ketamine is a dissociative anesthetic labeled for cats and nonhuman primates, but at one time it was widely used in humans. This was stopped because it caused nightmares.

The vet in LA told me about a vein that runs up the back of the calf in chimps. I would never have thought to look there.

A human anesthesiologist told me I couldn't just open up the intravenous line as I might do in a dog. Fluid overload is a real problem in humans, and it followed there could be a problem in a chimp, since Jeeter so resembled a human, both in appearance and biologically. I carefully figured the fastest safe infusion rate—I didn't want to keep him out long, but I wanted to rehydrate him as much as possible.

A local pediatrician gave me perhaps the most important tip of all. He told me about an antibiotic called Rocephin. This is a third-generation cephalosporin, a distant cousin of Keflex, available only by injection. It comes in a powder, and must be reconstituted with a local anesthetic if it is to be given intramuscularly, because it hurts so much. However, it is safe for intravenous injection, and—here's why it was such great news—

lasts twenty-four hours after it is given. It would not require dosing every eight hours like its cheaper cousin, cephazolin, which we used so much of at the emergency clinic.

A pharmacist at the hospital arranged for Dan to pick up three vials. Once it was mixed up, it had to be used quickly or it would lose efficacy.

While he went to pick up the medication, I laid out everything I would need. I drew up the ketamine—Dan would have to inject it into Jeeter's muscle. That was the weakest link in our plan. Once Jeeter was groggy from the injection, I would place a mask over his face and deliver a mixture of oxygen and isoflurane, until he was sufficiently under to allow a throat culture followed by endotracheal intubation. Then he would be maintained on isoflurane until we were finished.

I would place two catheters—one in each calf. If possible, I would use long jugular catheters, which might be harder for him to remove once he awoke. Once I had even one in place, we would commence the intravenous drip, the precious electrolyte solution that would add much-needed fluids to his body and deliver the medication once it was on board.

While the fluids were running, I would draw blood for a lab panel, to be sent to the human hospital by prior arrangement. I would place the second catheter, improving our chances of having one still in place the following day when we repeated the injection.

Last, we would wrap adhesive tape around each finger and toe. The object of this—a tip from the vet in Los Angeles—was to keep Jeeter distracted after he woke up. I wanted to be able to repeat the injection a day later without having to put him under again. That required a catheter to still be in place. Jeeter had hands. He would be more efficient at removing catheters than the most unruly dog had been. With luck he would spend his efforts removing the tape instead of the IV lines.

I went through the sequence several times in my mind. Dan's help would be crucial to the success of our plan, and he was a worried parent. I had to remain calm and pretend confidence, since I was afraid he would crumble.

Dan and Jeeter arrived. Simultaneously, so did a cat with an abscessed wound on his face. Dan waited in the Treatment room while I saw the cat. The cat was not happy when I deposited it in a cage within sight of the chimp, but it distracted Jeeter while Dan gave him the ketamine in his thigh. Ketamine hurts, and the expression on Jeeter's face after he received it was full of human hurt and betrayal. But he would not hurt Dan. I was grateful I hadn't had to give the shot myself. I had been worried Dan couldn't do it. He had, and now the rest was up to me.

Everything went exactly as planned. When Jeeter went home, still a bit sluggish but walking, I felt I had done all I could. I sent the samples off to the hospital hoping we hadn't missed something significant. The blood tests came back normal. The culture would take a few days.

On Sunday Jeeter definitely felt better. When he returned for his second treatment, I could see it in his movements. He was curious, more alert, freer in his gait.

And he had a total of two toes taped and one catheter still in place. I mixed up the injection and gave it into the catheter while Dan held Jeeter on the table. As I pushed the plunger on the syringe, Jeeter turned to look first at me—my heart leaped, but it was just a glance—then at the leg. His expression clearly said, "Where did *that* come from?" Even intravenously, apparently the stuff burned. Fingers reached for the tape holding the catheter in place. I finished the injection and flushed the line. He had it out before he got to the van.

But that was okay. It was enough. The culture eventually confirmed a strep infection, which was quite sensitive to the drug we had chosen. On the third day, Jeeter was stealing the other chimps' oatmeal, and willingly took his Keflex in food. He was back to his ornery self, only twice as hungry.

Jeeter's recovery involved the participation of two veterinarians, two pediatricians, a surgeon, an anesthesiologist, and a primate trainer. It brought a whole new meaning to the term "team approach to medicine."

A few days later I stopped by on my way home from work to see Jeeter. Dan had the garage door open, giving the chimps fresh air while he cleaned up their environment. He opened Jeeter's cage and—unlike when he was sick—allowed him to greet me.

Before I knew what was happening, I had my arms around a small ape, and he was hugging me with both his arms and his legs. When he felt well, Jeeter could be very affectionate.

Pigskin

"Do you treat potbellied pigs?"

"Not if I can help it. Tell them to call one of the equine vets."

"They tried that. No one's available."

"What's wrong with the pig?"

"It was attacked by three dogs. The owner says it's pretty torn up."

I sighed. My experience with pet pigs to date had not been rewarding. The first one was owned by a jerk who never brought his pet in until it was nearly dead, then stopped payment on his check. The next one was a baby that died despite heroic efforts to save its bacon, if you'll pardon the expression. That summed up my experience.

Still, how could I go wrong sewing up bite wounds?

"Okay, if she wants to bring it in, I'll see what I can do."

Hammy Faye Bacon was no ordinary pig. She was no miniature, either. Easily a hundred pounds, she was covered with bite wounds. Both ears had been torn off, and the skin around her neck was in strips. We hefted her into the tub and I tried to examine her. She dodged forward and back and squealed as if we were trying to eat her alive.

Of course, for all she knew, we were no different from the dogs who had done just that.

Somewhere I had an article on anesthesia in these guys. I tracked it down and discovered that, indeed, we had the required drugs on hand. I drew them up and gave the injection. And waited for them to take effect.

And waited.

After twenty minutes, she did seem quieter. But she wasn't

ready to let me sew her up yet. We got out the gas machine and masked her with isoflurane, on the theory that iso was the safest thing going. Another fifteen minutes and she was more or less still.

Pigskin isn't like other skin. It's thick and stiff and does not stretch or maneuver to cover open spaces. I found tags of tissue to sew to the remnants of her ear canals—after all, the outer pinnae are not necessary for hearing. Much of the shredded hide was dead and had to be removed. Covering the resulting open areas was an exercise in creative determination. She had gashes along both flanks and her back as well. I sutured diligently, using extra-heavy suture. Eventually everything came together, more or less. It took almost three hours.

I've seen dogs die from shock after suffering less extensive wounds. Hammy Faye Bacon had seemed quite tolerant of whatever degree of pain she felt, but losing that much skin had to take its toll. I had no means of giving fluids—normally I would have used an ear vein. I did inject dexamethasone for the swelling and to help protect against shock, and of course started aggressive antibiotic therapy—at least I hoped so, given my lack of knowledge of swine doses. I sent more home for her owner to inject twice a day. I was not optimistic.

She woke up uneventfully. Any other animal I would have hospitalized, but since there was little I could do in case of a crisis, and I really didn't have the facilities to keep a pig, I sent this one home.

I called the next night to check on her. "She's hanging in there," her owner said. "She ate as soon as she got home." That was always a good sign. "She's moving a little stiffly but otherwise she looks good!"

Two days later the sutures were still holding. If she'd survived that long, her odds were quite good. "And she can hear!" her owner reported. "I called her over for dinner, when I was standing behind her. And she turned around and came over!"

I never saw Hammy Faye again (eventually the sutures would have dissolved on their own). I don't know if she was representative of the species, but her resilience was amazing. The very image of an earless pig, the wrinkles stretched out of her skin and a crazy quilt of stitches running over her body, has stayed with me.

I suppose one could say that Hammy Faye Bacon had gotten the face-lift of a lifetime!

Sara Howls

The first time I met Virginia Skinner, she brought me a coyote to treat.

At the time, Virginia was the veterinarian at the Living Desert, our local zoo. Sara, the coyote, was nine years old and had been at the zoo all her life. She wasn't exactly tame, but she knew her keeper and trusted her. She was one of the most popular attractions there—she lived alone in her pen, but when children passed by and howled, she would answer. The cries—human and coyote—reverberated throughout the compound. The normally nocturnal creature seemed to enjoy the attention. Perhaps the children entertained her as much as she did them.

For reasons we never understood, Sara's temperature had suddenly shot up to 109 degrees Fahrenheit. Normal would be the same as a dog's—around 102. The extreme fever caused a reaction in her brain resulting in sudden and complete blindness.

Not wanting to leave her alone, and definitely wanting a second opinion, Virginia and the Living Desert management decided to bring her to the emergency clinic for overnight monitoring. Virginia and the keeper carried her in in a large dog crate. We had to drag her out with a rabies pole around her neck. It broke my heart to see this terrified, blind, wild creature, delirious with fever, fighting, she assumed, for her life against that pole. We went over her, got an IV in and injected her with various medications, then ensconced her in a run. Virginia and the keeper left.

I was not optimistic. She was thin and hot. She was not young. The fever's cause was never determined. Lab work was normal. We treated her with fluids, antibiotics, and antipyretics. She did not begin to trust us. Her vision showed no sign of returning even as her temperature came down. Could a blind coyote manage, even in a zoo? No one knew.

But Sara was tougher than we suspected. She never recovered her vision, but lived to be fifteen. She had a smallish enclosed pen all to herself.

And until the day she died, when the children howled, Sara howled back.

An Act
Of Courage

One quiet night Palm Springs Police Department's dispatcher called. An officer was bringing in a vicious dog. She didn't say why they were bringing it to us, so we prepared for the worst.

She arrived at the end of a rabies pole. She was an emaciated, filthy mess, a pit bull who was probably white beneath the filth. Her mammary glands hung nearly to the floor, and were full. There was a litter of puppies somewhere that belonged to her.

She looked to be young—maybe two or three. I doubted she'd ever had a bath in her life, or a vaccination. It was equally unlikely this was her first litter of puppies.

She stood in the exam room, head hung miserably, the snare just allowing her to breathe. Expecting abuse. She'd learned not to fight back.

I crouched near her, not looking directly at her, and spoke gently. She may not have understood the words, but dogs always respond to tone. I spoke to the burly police officer at the other end of the pole.

"Is she injured?" I couldn't see any sign of it, but I hadn't really gotten close enough to look.

"I don't think so. She attacked us when we went to arrest her owner. He's a crack dealer and a small-time pimp." He told me where she'd come from. Even Palm Springs has its crime-infested neighborhood.

About then my hand made contact with the dog. She tensed, then her tail moved in a tentative wag. Her neck was still extended in front of her. She didn't move a muscle.

"Her eyes are closed, like there's something wrong there," I said in the same even tone.

"That's pepper spray. Be sure and wash your hands before you touch your face."

My heart sank. This poor wretched creature lived half-starved and appeared not to know how to accept affection. She'd tried to protect the creep who owned her, or her puppies, or both. The police officers, already adrenaline-charged just from being in the area, had reacted correctly. But I wished it hadn't happened.

By now she was relaxing as I rubbed her ears, scratched the back of her neck. The tail moved in a small, almost apologetic arc as I convinced her no one was going to hurt her if she didn't hurt us. I loosened the snare and she didn't budge.

"Where are her puppies?" I asked.

"We'll go back and get them tomorrow."

Sharon and I exchanged glances. "They probably won't make it that long."

That was all I said about it. I wasn't about to suggest these policemen risk their lives a second time to rescue a litter of pit bull puppies that would most likely just be put to sleep anyway.

But that's just what they did. It was over an hour later, and they'd had to send two units. They'd had to enter that house, where other residents still lived, and remove six two-week-old puppies so they wouldn't starve. The same officer presented them to the little bitch, who by now had endured a soapy bath, had her eyes flushed copiously, consumed two cans of high-calorie food, and was working on some kibble.

She stopped eating when she saw the puppies. For the first time she really wagged her tail. She looked directly at the officer who had sprayed pepper in her eyes, and she wagged her tail. As we placed the puppies in her cage, she licked each one and made no move to threaten anyone.

Animal Control picked her up the next morning. I don't know for sure what happened to her and those six pups. I have made it a point not to ask, because I probably would not like the answer. The bitch had attacked a police officer. She could not be returned to her owner, and she could not be adopted out. The puppies might have been bottle-raised, and perhaps they all found homes. The correct thing—the *legal* thing—to do was put them all to sleep. But I'd like to think a few of them slipped through and were adopted into loving homes.

Those officers knew all that when they went back to that house and rescued those puppies. They went anyway. Because it was the *humane* thing to do.

We dealt with PSPD on many occasions, and they were always professional and conscientious. But in my mind that single act spoke volumes. I'll always admire them for not letting those puppies starve to death.

Whodunit?

Rarely did a day go by that I was not asked to euthanize someone's pet. Normally this decision is one the owner has reached after agonizing thought, and the final injection is a service to both human and animal. The pet is dying or suffering in a way that either cannot be alleviated, or is beyond the means of its owner. Occasionally, however, the request is made for murkier reasons.

Sometimes I refuse. I am under no obligation to provide such a service simply because someone asks. However, in the case where a dog has bitten a human, or attacked another animal viciously and without provocation, I may agree. But the decision to euthanize a healthy animal is one that must be considered with excruciating care. No case has ever illustrated this point to me as clearly as "Willie" Jones.

Willie's owner had visitors. An adult daughter, Vanessa, her husband Jim and two children, and the family's two dogs had come for a week. The dogs—a big terrier named Rascal and a mutt called Boo, who obviously had some pit bull in his makeup—seemed to get along with Willie and his "brother," a shepherd-cross dubbed Waylon. So the extended family felt comfortable leaving them all together while the humans went out to dinner.

Willie was not a youngster. In fact, at sixteen, he may have been one of the oldest English setters in the world. Nevertheless, he got along in life. His day consisted of breakfast, a trip through the doggy door to the backyard to "do his business," then back inside for a nap. This nap often lasted until dinner, at which time the pattern was repeated. Except in the evening he preferred to nap outside.

This particular night was warm but windy. The Jones family

lived in Cathedral City, on the edge abutting open desert. It's an area where wind is a frequent visitor, even the tearing dust storms that had gusted the entire desert over the past several days. Willie tottered outside as usual that evening for his sleep.

The yard was fenced. In fact, it was surrounded by a five-foot cement-block wall, which was nearly new and in excellent repair.

But the Jones family returned home to find Waylon, Rascal, and Boo inside, very agitated. They anxiously led the Joneses to the doggy door. Upon investigating, they found Willie in the yard, comatose, with severe lacerations over his neck, hindquarters, and one side. The wounds were not only deep, but had sand and dried grass ground into them, a surgeon's nightmare. Willie was nearly dead.

When I first saw him, I thought: *coyotes.* These predators thrive in the desert, frequently impinging on neighborhoods in search of food. A coyote is a wild animal, and would as soon eat a pet as the pet's food. They have a characteristic way of attacking: One pack member goes for the throat while another snares the hind legs. In Willie's case pieces of muscle were actually missing. Whoever had done this meant business.

But no, the Joneses assured me. No coyote could get over their wall. It must have been the other dogs.

With a heavy heart I set about stabilizing Willie. His body temperature had plummeted due to shock, and I had no idea how much of the shredded skin would be salvageable. Infection was likely to be severe. Fortunately, there were good veins and I set about pumping volumes of warmed electrolyte solution into him. I lavaged his lacerations and covered them with sterile wet dressing, hoping to preserve as much tissue as possible for surgery the following day. I transfused him as soon as his temperature started coming up. He regained consciousness and I treated his pain. But he was not ready for anesthesia and surgery to repair his wounds that night.

It was a long night for Willie. It was a long night for the Joneses, as well.

"We've decided to have you put Rascal and Boo to sleep," Vanessa told me the next morning.

I understood their reasoning. I asked them to think it over first. Grimly they conveyed Willie to their regular vets, Doug

Kunz and Garry Roberts, for the day. I felt sure that if anyone could sew Willie back together and make it stick, these folks could do it.

It must have taken hours. But when he returned that evening, Willie's awful wounds were closed. And the Joneses all looked better. They had some good news to impart.

They'd thought about what I said the night before. They'd gone outside that day and walked around the yard. Though any tracks had been obliterated, the wind had blown piles of sand against the wall—the outside on the east wall, the inside on the west. And caught in a tiny crevice on the wall's rounded top was a tuft of brown fur.

Coyote fur.

The loose sand was high enough to enable the coyotes to jump the wall to get in. Spotting Willie lying there asleep, old and apparently alone, they'd seen an easy meal.

Boo and Rascal didn't attack Willie, they saved him.

The Dog
That Wouldn't Die

Since long before I attended vet school, reliable euthanasia compounds have been routinely available to veterinarians. Nowadays the norm is pentobarbital—an overdose of a drug that was once used for anesthesia, but has been replaced in that duty by safer protocols.

But ask someone who's been in the profession a little longer—say, since the year I was born—and chances are he'll have at least one story to tell about euthanasia gone wrong. This one was told to me by a member of the Emergency Clinic's board of directors, whom I will refer to as Dr. X, and it took place in the early 1960s.

It seems Dr. X had a patient with a large tumor on its abdomen. I'll call the dog Bones, though I have no idea what its real name was. This was long before chemotherapy was widely available even for humans, and this tumor was much too large to remove, at least on the budget available to Bones's owners. At ten, Bones was considered an old dog, and they didn't want to put him through surgery. (How things have changed!)

The growth was becoming unsightly, however, and beginning to embarrass his owners. So they decided the only thing to do was to have their pet put to sleep. Having made the decision, they conveyed the dog to Dr. X, explained what they wanted, and left him at the clinic, confident that Bones would be gone by closing time.

Now, DVMs have always enjoyed a reputation for being frugal—okay, cheap—and this one was no exception. Before laws were passed to regulate such things, it was considered acceptable to use expired anesthetic drugs as euthanasia agents. Since the anesthetics of the day were notoriously unpredictable, it was a simple matter to give a moderate overdose to induce quick, painless—and usually efficient—death.

And that's exactly what Dr. X did.

Another thing that's changed is the method of disposal of animal carcasses. Today most are buried or cremated. In the sixties, however, the veterinarian commonly transported the bodies to the town dump, which were simpler affairs themselves—none of the constant digging and leveling that goes on today.

So Dr. X dropped his presumedly deceased patient at the dump on his way home that evening.

Two days later the owners received a telephone call. A man who had gone to the dump looking for salvageable objects had found a dog wandering among the trash. The dog had a collar on, and on the collar were his license and rabies tags. Being an animal lover, he had contacted town hall and been given the owners' names—again, before the Privacy Act. He looked them up in the phone book and told them he had their dog, which he had found at the town dump.

Obviously—to me, and to Dr. X—what happened was this: The unstable anesthetic agent had deteriorated somewhat after expiration, and instead of death merely induced a very deep plane of anesthesia. The dog slept, maybe for a day or two, only to wake up confused and no doubt ravenously hungry. Finding himself at the dump, he began foraging for something to eat, whereupon the nice man found him and eventually contacted his owners.

The owners, however, had been having second thoughts. They missed their pet and wondered if they hadn't been hasty in their decision. The mass, after all, didn't seem to bother the dog much. It just looked funny. They had been earnestly praying for reassurance that they had done the right thing.

The phone call was, for them, a clear case of divine intervention.

Bones lived another two years, and died in his sleep—apparently of old age.

Where There's Smokey
There's Fire

Police agencies from various desert cities brought us patients from time to time. But this was the first time I could recall the Fire Department doing so.

They brought us two cats in a cardboard box. They reeked of smoke. They were charcoal-colored from the soot clinging to their fur. They hissed up at me, showing pink gums and gleaming eyes—the only parts that reflected light. After smoke and flames had invaded their domain, then water and strangers, and after being stuffed into a box and taken for an unexpected ride, they didn't trust anyone.

I slid them into the incubator, oxygen running full-force, and examined them through the Plexiglas. I'd half-expected severe burns when the call came in, but these guys were just breathing a little hard. Smoke inhalation was the biggest concern. And both had burned the pads of all four feet and their noses. Their once-lush fur had insulated them from the worst of the heat. They resented my touching them, and were able to stand, at least in a crouch, so I left them alone for the time being.

"Is the owner all right?" I asked, assuming she was or they wouldn't have bothered with the cats.

"We have no idea."

That got my attention. "What?"

"She wasn't home. It was an apartment fire. Looks like pretty obvious arson."

"You think she set it herself? With her cats in the house?" I sincerely hoped that wasn't the case.

"We don't really know. One of the neighbors said she'd been fighting with her boyfriend. I've got to go."

Since we didn't have an account with the Fire Department,

and the city in question always resisted paying for animal treatment, I had a bit of a dilemma on my hands. Their owner, who was now homeless, might not be able to keep the cats anymore. She might not want to spend her money treating them. There's nothing worse than getting an animal through a crisis only to have it put down just when it was getting better, simply because no one wants it.

Fortunately, the cats weren't too badly injured, but they still needed treatment. I decided they could handle the steroids to help protect their lungs, and an antibiotic injection each to guard against pneumonia. And, what the heck, a little painkiller didn't cost that much. I'd have liked to put them on IVs but we were getting into much more involved care there. As long as they appeared stable, I'd keep them on oxygen and wait to hear from their owner.

Beneath the soot, one of the cats seemed to have been gray, the other black. "I guess we'll call them Smokey and Charcoal," Sharon said.

I groaned but was laughing, too. Our sense of humor could get a little weird sometimes.

"Well, we have to call them something." The cats themselves just seemed to want to be left alone. They huddled together with their eyes shut. We put antibiotic ointment in their eyes and left them to rest.

It was well after midnight when the owner finally called. Her name was Shana. She'd returned home from a nightclub, where she'd been partying with a friend, to find her apartment burned and drenched, the door hanging open and her cats nowhere to be found. It had taken frantic phone calls to 911 and the Fire Department, and some awakened neighbors, to get the story.

It was now my unpleasant duty to tell this distraught young woman that I needed a guarantee of payment before I could further treat the cats. "We're probably looking at a few hundred dollars each," I said. "I'm most concerned about their lungs, and it's too early to tell how bad the damage is. The good news is that cats are small and smoke rises, so they would have been underneath the worst of it."

"So you think they'll be okay?" The shock was apparent in her voice.

"Yeah, I think they will. But I don't *know*."

"Well, I guess . . . go ahead and treat them. Can I leave them there for a few days?"

That seemed fair. I asked her to come down the next morning or evening to fill out some paperwork, got a phone number for the friend she would be staying with, and was about to hang up. "Oh, wait a sec! What are their names?"

"The cats? Smokey and Soot."

I didn't speak for a moment. Then, "You're kidding."

Shana laughed, and I admired her for being able to see the humor. "No, and I was thinking about taking in another one. She's a red tabby and I was gonna name her Flame."

I burst out laughing. I couldn't help it. "Maybe you ought to reconsider," was all I could reply.

"Yeah, you're probably right."

The cats did fine. The bill was less than predicted.

Shana picked them up a couple of days later. Once they'd settled down we had bathed them, but they still smelled of smoke. Their feet were bandaged, their eyes were bright, and they were breathing evenly. Their burned noses were islands of pink in otherwise monochrome faces.

Shana had arranged to move in with another friend for a few months until she got back on her feet. Most of her clothes and some of the furniture had survived the fire, which apparently had been concentrated in the living room. A former boyfriend had set the fire and been arrested. Apparently he'd arrived at her apartment unannounced and found her gone. In a drunken rage, he'd set fire to some paper and pushed it under the door.

"Thanks for taking care of them," she said as she picked up their carriers—soot-scented survivors of the fire. "I'm changing their names, though. From now on they're gonna be Lucky and Bum."

I'm sure the cats didn't mind.

Cuts
Like A Knife

It's hard to tell, sometimes, how seriously injured an animal is based on its owner's demeanor. I've had children screaming—and parents, too, for that matter—over torn toenails, painful ears, anything over which a bit of melodrama may be mustered. One woman, forced to wait with her injured dog while we saw others who had arrived ahead of her, repeatedly insisted that her pet must see the doctor "immediately, before she bleeds to death!" As evidence, she displayed the tissue she had been using to dab at a nearly invisible wound on the dog's side. The tissue, far from soaked, was tinged a slight pink after fifteen minutes or so of this persistent dabbing. Jane at the front desk told her, straight-faced, to stop dabbing at the wound or the doctor would have trouble locating it.

On the other hand, because they don't understand the anatomy and are usually responding to the animal's degree of excitement or amount of visible blood, some of the most severely injured pets are brought in by remarkably calm owners. "I think something is wrong," or "He was grabbed by a big dog last night and I think he's got a cut on one side," are fairly frequent complaints, as they bundle the pet under one arm and sit to quietly fill out the information sheet and wait their turn. I once walked into an exam room to see a cyanotic Yorkie, weak from shock and lack of oxygen, lying against the table in a way that saved his life—he had a sucking chest wound which had not been evident to the owner because of the long, matted hair that covered it. The stainless steel table now sealed the wound completely.

When a chest wall is perforated, every breath pulls air into the chest cavity through the skin, instead of into the lungs. When ribs are broken, as was the case for this Yorkie, the pain leads to shallow breathing, which just makes things worse. The result is rapid loss of oxygen from the bloodstream, and death.

Like many of his breed, this one was moderately overweight. His fat had partially filled the defect and allowed a semblance of intact thoracic wall. The dog survived, but I've often wondered how it got to me alive. That one, at least, had a history compatible with his injuries—he had been grabbed by a German shepherd and shaken, and the owners saw the whole thing.

Once in a while, however, I saw injuries with no explanation whatsoever. Since cats are wanderers, it's easier to guess how one might have crawled into the neighbor's truck's engine to take a nap and been cut by the fan when the neighbor left for work the next morning. Or mauled by a dog, or beaten up by another cat, or even struck by a car—a fate less often survived by cats than dogs. With a little practice and observation, one notices indicators—toenails frayed when a cat clutches the pavement, the pattern of punctures associated with another cat's claws.

But with dogs, confined to a fenced yard or even leash walks, some lacerations seem inexplicable. I've seen large gashes that appear to be the result of a glancing blow from a sharp object, enormous sticks of wood nearly imbedded in muscle, deep abscesses with no apparent puncture at all.

And then there was Charlie.

Charlie was a mutt. Mixed breed, all-American . . . whatever. Black-and-white and nondescript, he waited in the car while his owner, a reasonable calm woman, entered the clinic and said, "My dog has a cut on his side. I don't think he can walk in and he's too big for me to carry."

Jane gave her the form to fill out, and she did so. Sharon got the stretcher and the two of us accompanied Barbara LaShantz to her car.

Charlie stood between the front and rear seats, leaning against the upright backrest with an anxious expression on his face.

"I think it's on the side you can't see," Ms. LaShantz said. The sight of her dog seemed to make her more distraught.

I climbed into the car to give the dog a quick going-over. "Hey, Charlie. Good boy. Good Charlie." One never knows how a dog will react to having his car invaded, but Charlie either didn't mind or knew he couldn't do anything about it. I rubbed his ears so my first touch would not be a painful one, then worked my way back. The fingers of my right hand slipped between him and the seat back and between two ribs and into a void. The dog's concern visibly increased.

I backed out, holding my bloody hand out. I was stunned. "He's got an enormous laceration in his left chest wall. I don't know how he got here alive."

He was leaning against the seats, breathing okay for now. We stood there for a bit while I formulated a plan. Finally Sharon carried the stretcher back inside and returned with a roll of plastic wrap—ordinary kitchen wrap. I pulled a long piece off and wrapped it around Charlie's chest to seal the wound, then lifted him and carried him quickly into the back room.

Charlie wore no collar. He was not neutered. Ms. LaShantz had skipped the part of the questionnaire that asked about the dog's vaccination history. He was a nice dog, but I suspected he was an afterthought in the family hierarchy. I covered the wound more thoroughly, hoping I was not merely subjecting him to more discomfort before being asked to finish the job someone else had started. I did not think the cost for what was needed was within this client's reach.

Once more layers of plastic were in place, I addressed Charlie's owner. "This looks like a knife wound. What happened?"

She was beginning to crumble. "I don't know. He just went outside like he always does, and he never came back. I went out and found him like this."

"He was in your yard?" I asked, trying to imagine what sort of protrusion or debris might cause a wound like this—and failing to picture it.

"Not exactly," she admitted. "There's this place where the fence is sort of . . . where it doesn't really meet, in one corner? He squeezes through there sometimes."

I was getting frustrated, wishing she would just tell me what had happened so I could understand what I was dealing with. I knew it was a shock for her, too. I admired her for keeping herself together this long. But I needed information. "So he was outside the fence?"

"Yeah."

"Are there any sharp points where the fencing might have cut him?" But the laceration went too deep for that, surely.

"Nuh-no." She was hugging herself and appeared cold despite the July desert heat. Sharon turned the air-conditioning down but I doubted that would help.

"What's behind the fence?" I asked gently. It seemed important to learn as much as possible before she fell apart completely.

"It's just the alley. Sometimes kids hang out back there. He likes to bark at them."

That's the most I ever learned. That Charlie, either wanting to play or defending his territory, climbed through the break in the fence and was knifed by a young terrorist. Ms. LaShantz had not heard barking or suspected a problem—so she said—until she went outside to find her dog standing in the alley unable to move. I never learned who picked him up and carried him to the car. The dog needed surgery, and his owner either could or could not afford it. I put it to her bluntly.

She said she could. "Of course, we have to treat him!" she said. "I have kids!"

She gave Jane a credit card. Sharon and I set up for emergency surgery and began shock treatment. Amazingly, despite the depth of the wound, transfusion was not required. But I knew we would be working on Charlie for quite a while.

An open chest meant Sharon had to do Charlie's breathing for him. We moved quickly and had him on the table within forty minutes of his arrival. For the first time I saw the true extent of the laceration.

It had to have been a knife, and the stabbing deliberate. The wound margins were too clean, too deep for it to have been anything else. The laceration appeared to move from midway up the dog's side, upwards, severing two ribs from the spine and slicing into the muscles of his back. My fingers, probing the muscle tear, stopped against bone. "If the little psychopath had paid attention in biology class, this dog would be dead," I said bitterly. "It's pure luck he missed the heart."

"Or lousy aim," Sharon put in.

"Either way." I stitched muscle. Sharon inflated his lungs.

It was a clean wound, and he was a shorthaired dog, so there was little visible contamination. Still, in between breaths I had Sharon gently pour warmed saline into the chest cavity to lavage out the small stuff I couldn't see. Charlie was very fortunate in that his mediastinum—the thick band of tissue that separates the two halves of the thorax—was intact, so that when he tried to breathe he was able to move some air even with half his chest nonfunctional.

By repairing the tissue on either side of the severed ribs, I was able to stabilize them pretty well. Then I moved on to the intercostal muscle, the layer between ribs that formed the longest segment of the wound. As I sewed I reflected that, not so long ago, I had not possessed the surgical skill to repair this dog's chest. That scared me, too, because the technical skills were not that demanding. It was the terrifying idea of working in the chest cavity that might easily have intimidated me into putting the dog to sleep.

I think then I realized that many *would* have euthanized Charlie. They would not have been wrong to do so. His was a time-consuming case, and the potential for complications was extremely high. But this was exactly the sort of case the emergency clinic existed to treat. With no small sense of accomplishment I started in sewing skin.

Charlie had a chest tube for two days. He was walking the morning after surgery. Despite pain medication, he moved carefully—but I saw no evidence of severe nerve damage or postoperative bleeding.

The bill approached two thousand dollars by the time Charlie went home. His owner's credit card maxed out at around a thousand. We held postdated checks for the rest. The first two cleared without incident. After that—and long after the sutures had been removed and Charlie resumed normal activities—the next check came back stamped "ACCOUNT CLOSED." Letters requesting payment were returned undeliverable. When Jane tried to add the balance to the credit card number she still held in reserve, it was declined.

The account went to collection, but the agency never located the LaShantz family. I want to believe the woman intended to pay her bill but fell on hard times. I don't know where they moved to, but I hope their new house has an intact fence and a big yard for Charlie to play in.

Moving On

I worked at Animal Emergency Clinic of the Desert for six years before I realized it would not be my lifelong career. The irregular schedule, erratic staffing, and constant awareness of the fact that I often could not please the clients, the board, and the referring veterinarians all at the same time, all contributed to my decision. Add to that the unpredictability of each day—the very thing I used to thrive on—and I just got tired.

I understand that, statistically speaking, MDs who choose emergency work have a practice life expectancy roughly half that of other specialties before they burn out and either leave the profession, change specialties, or move into administration. If similar statistics exist for veterinarians it would not surprise me. I noticed that a large percentage of those I knew who had worked emergency for several years were also getting out of it.

For years the excitement and professional challenge of the emergency room were enough to overshadow my desire to own my own practice. I knew I could manage a practice well, and I liked the idea of a small clinic with one or two employees.

One thing emergency practice did not allow was case follow-up. For years that was a nuisance but not something I gave a lot of thought to. It turns out I was missing a lot.

It took me two years to hire a replacement for myself and extract myself from the regular schedule there. In the meantime I located an excellent clinic site in a shopping center in Palm Desert, and with the help of my friend and attorney Joan Baumgarten, negotiated a lease. That process and the build-out took over a year. I opened Country Club Animal Clinic on August 1, 1996. I had one employee, Kitty Flanders, and it was my lucky day indeed when she applied for the job.

My overhead is high; I started with the very best I could afford, both in equipment and location. I have only myself and my clients to please—and if a client is especially unreasonable I now have the luxury of inviting them to take their pets elsewhere. (So far I haven't had to do this, because all my clients are delightful—but it's nice to know I can!)

But it was hard letting go. I still have to fight against calling Jane, to offer advice. I now sympathize with the local vets who tended to go over my head to the board when they were unhappy with something that happened under my management. I've come close to doing the same thing.

What goes around comes around, I guess. I'm very happy with my laid-back practice, and it's already growing. Already I have a second staff member, Kathy Ross—who used to work for Dr. Vicki Robertson. Kitty left and I hired two people to replace her—a full-time technician, Lisa Penault, and a part-time assistant, Barbara Mathes. Eventually I will expand my hours, hire more staff and a second veterinarian. But for now I'm very content for things to remain as they are.

I never intended to make the desert my home.

As is often said, sometimes life is what happens while we're busy making plans.

Mr. Gilmore's
Kitten

He lay in the supermarket parking lot in a box, weak and cold and abandoned. About five months old, with long gray-and-white fur, he gazed bleakly back at his rescuers.

This was a kitten who knew about people. No feral-born stray, he was clean and well-fed and very affectionate. He had belonged to someone. He had probably gotten outside and been hit by a car, and his owners were unable or unwilling to pay for veterinary services. So they dumped him in the parking lot of a supermarket in an affluent part of town.

He was discovered by employees of the supermarket just as Stuart Gilmore was getting out of his car to buy groceries. Mr. Gilmore had lost two geriatric cats over the previous year, both to complications of kidney failure, and had been on the lookout for a new one. He accepted the box, got back in his old station wagon, and rushed across the street to Nancy Carlson's office. She was closer than my newly opened clinic, and it was Thursday, the day I closed early.

It was almost too late. The kitten's body temperature had fallen to 96 degrees. His gums were pale, and a blood count confirmed severe anemia, though the cause was not apparent. One femur—the long bone extending from the hip to the stifle, or knee—was broken at the growth plate, and it looked as if he might have a broken pelvis as well.

"He's in pretty bad shape," Nancy told him.

"Please do everything you can to save him." That was Mr. Gilmore's way. He wasn't a wealthy man, but he loved cats. If one of his cats had any chance of surviving, he denied it nothing. And from the moment he saw it in that basket in the parking lot, this gray-and-white fluff ball became one of his cats. He'd already named it Muffin by the time he arrived at Nancy's.

The kitten was strong enough to fight when her staff took the X-rays, so Nancy was optimistic.

Nancy's staff started an IV, and began warming the kitten with warm IV fluids and a heating pad. Within hours it was purring and eating baby food. That was a Thursday, so Nancy planned to stabilize him and surgically repair the leg the following Monday.

Muffin did well until Friday night, at which time he stopped eating. Saturday his gums were paler, and his heart had begun a bizarre rhythm called a "gallop" rhythm, because, instead of the usual lub-*dup*, lub-*dup*, you hear a three-beat score not unlike the sound of a single horse galloping on a hard surface. He was laboring to breathe, and his pale gums had taken on a bluish cast.

That's how he was when I first saw him. Muffin was transferred to the Emergency Clinic for the weekend. I was still working there, a shift or two per week, supplementing the meager income from my fledgling practice until they could hire a second veterinarian.

Chest X-rays revealed bruises in Muffin's lungs. Though an electrocardiogram appeared normal, Muffin was presumed to have cardiac contusions, or bruises in his heart muscle, which often don't show up as a problem until several days after the trauma that causes them. The extent of the damage was unclear, so we could not predict what would happen. Mr. Gilmore, now obviously depressed, asked us again to do everything possible.

First, we drew blood to check the kitten for feline leukemia virus, feline immunodeficiency virus, and feline infectious peritonitis virus. He was negative for all three, so the cause of his medical problems was most likely related to the trauma that had broken his leg.

By this time Muffin was in our incubator, receiving oxygen. Since he had stopped eating and was so anemic, I slipped a tiny tube through his nose into his stomach and began feeding him a liquid diet in hopes of boosting his strength and his red cell volume without a transfusion. He lay limply in the incubator, no longer purring but responding with a squint when his cheek was rubbed.

He reminded me of all that I missed about emergency work.

That night his lungs began filling with edema fluid, a sign that the heart wasn't doing its job. We reduced the rate our fluids entered his body, so that now he was getting only a few milliliters per hour. And I started him on heart medicine—Lasix and captopril, drugs to reduce the burden on the heart by lowering blood pressure—therapies one associates with old dogs with loud heart murmurs and hacking coughs. Late-stage, salvaging therapies. But at least it helped the kitten breathe.

All that night I debated whether to give the little guy a transfusion. Every time I tripped over one of the clinic cats (there were now three, and Tex had retired as a donor), I thought about it. But so far his hematocrit held steady, though only about fifteen percent, a good ten points below normal. Each time I thought about it, I decided to wait.

Sunday morning he was a little better. He responded more attentively, lay sternal instead of flat on his side, and occasionally watched what went on around his Plexiglas bubble. And, most significantly, the heart rhythm had returned to almost normal. It looked as if the battle was on its way to being won. Laurel Cain—the clinic's new director—came on duty at ten A.M., and I went home to sleep.

And the kitten began to fade again. That afternoon, his hematocrit dropped to eleven percent. His breathing was more labored than ever. Laurel increased his Lasix dose and gave Muffin the blood transfusion I'd kept putting off. The improvement was immediate and gratifying. The bill for Muffin's weekend stay made me wince, but Mr. Gilmore did not complain. When he transferred his new kitten to my clinic Monday morning, he was smiling for the first time in days.

Not having the commercial liquid diet to put down Muffin's tube, I walked down to Ralph's grocery for some goat milk. I never had to put it down the tube at all, as Muffin started eating that morning. He took only a little at first, but it was a definite step in the right direction. That afternoon his purr returned full-force.

Monday night was his last at the emergency clinic. Tuesday morning we stopped the heart medication altogether. When I told Mr. Gilmore the kitten didn't have to return to the emergency clinic that night, I think it was the first time he really believed the kitten would make it.

All week Muffin ate, as if making up for missed meals. He gained weight and purred and tried to walk on his bad leg. I had been afraid to put him under anesthesia, but I knew something had to be done about the leg before long, or the callus that formed at the fracture site would make it impossible to get it straight. The break was too high to bandage, and each time he tried to put weight on the leg he added trauma to the soft tissues in the area.

Coincidentally, a little rhesus monkey named Sandy had been bitten severely by Jeeter the chimp early that same week. Knowing she would need a skin graft, I had arranged for a traveling surgeon named Jim Felts to come to my clinic to do the repair. He would do it that Friday. And as long as he was in the neighborhood, he'd be glad to fix Muffin's leg.

The procedure went well. Though well over a week had passed since the initial trauma, almost no callus had formed. This was probably due to the fact that Muffin's body had been busy with his heart and lung travails, and there had not been enough oxygen or calories available to try to repair the leg. Because the break was so near a joint, Jim was far better qualified than I to do the job, and he quickly stacked three pins through the delicate bone. Muffin woke up ravenous and spent Friday night and Saturday at the emergency clinic, receiving pain medication as needed. I worked that Saturday, and Muffin could have been any healthy kitten. Except, that is, for the long row of sutures down the outside of one hind leg, and his tendency to slide rather than walk.

The expression on Mr. Gilmore's face the next morning as he carried Muffin to his car reminded me of what veterinary medicine is all about.

I saw the kitten several times over the next few weeks, for suture removal and more X-rays. He developed a large patch of dead skin near the original fracture site, and that had to be cut away. I neutered him while he was under.

Several weeks later he was back in the clinic with a sudden high fever. Blood work was normal, but he lay limply on the floor of his cage, reminding me so much of the days after he was found. I could not find a reason for the fever. I worried about a virus that had somehow escaped detection initially—the tests aren't perfect. But he still tested negative, and over the next twenty-four hours responded well to fluids and antibiotics. The next morning his appetite returned with a vengeance, and he went home purring and unconcerned. I don't know what made him sick, or if he'll get sick again in the future. But for now he's one lucky kitten, in a house full of lucky cats.

And a reminder of all the reasons I love daytime practice.

Read the entire
Andi Pauling mystery series

by

Lillian M. Roberts

"Roberts is one new writer who delivers
with the expertise of a veteran."
—Roderick Thorp

"Every animal lover wants a vet like Dr.
Andi Pauling with her cool analytical mind
and unfailingly warm heart."
—Martha C. Lawrence
Author of *Murder in Scorpio*

Published by Fawcett Books.
Available at your local bookstore.

RIDING FOR A FALL

The return of Ross McRoberts—an old flame from vet school—spells trouble for Andi Pauling's fledgling business.

First his horses become the targets of malicious sabotage, and then a popular Argentine polo player turns up dead . . .

Published by Fawcett Books.
Available at your local bookstore.

THE HAND THAT FEEDS YOU

Palm Springs vet Andi Pauling fears the worst when a client brings a severely battered pit bull to her for treatment.

Even more disturbing is the mute, withdrawn little girl accompanying him. When the dog's owner is murdered and the child vanishes, Andi infiltrates the nightmare world of the illegal dogfight circuit to find the girl—and becomes fair game for a vicious pack of very human predators.

Published by Fawcett Books.
Available at your local bookstore.

ALMOST HUMAN

Palm Springs vet Andi Pauling was accustomed to putting pets to sleep when their condition was hopeless—a sad but necessary procedure.

But she was unprepared for a pet owner's request to do the same for her. When the woman dies under suspicious circumstances, Andi finds herself in deep trouble—suspected of murder, and a target of vicious attacks. . . .

Published by Fawcett Books.
Available at your local bookstore.